KNOCKED OFF MY KNEES

Coping When Chronic Illness Hits Hard

Grace Casselman

PublishAmerica
Baltimore

First printing

ISBN: 1-59286-693-X
PUBLISHED BY PUBLISHAMERICA BOOK PUBLISHERS
www.publishamerica.com
Baltimore

Printed in the United States of America

To my husband Douglas, my stalwart bulwark.

And to my son Adam, my inspiration.

Index

The Weaver

My Life is but a weaving
Between my God and me;
I do not choose the colours
He works steadily.

Sometimes He weaves sorrow
And I, in foolish pride,
Forget He sees the upper,
And I the under side.

Not 'till the loom is silent
And the shuttles cease to fly,
Will God unroll the canvas
And explain the reason why.

The dark threads are as needful
In the Weaver's skillful hand,
As the threads of gold and silver
In the pattern He has planned.

Grant Colfax Tullar — American hymnist, 1869-1950

Foreword
by Dr. Henry Schorr

Senior Minister,
Centre Street Church,
Calgary, Alberta

Deep down inside us, there's the awareness that our lives are quite precarious.

We know that disease can strike, accidents can happen. We know that, but we do everything we can to push that reality out of our minds. In an affluent, peaceful society, we can often convince ourselves that we're really quite in control of our lives.

Bad things happen to other people, but we're pretty sure that we're secure, that we're insulated, that we're safe — these things won't happen to us. When we live free from calamity for long periods of time, not only do we feel a kind of invincibility, we start to take life itself for granted.

We start taking God for granted, we become more and more obsessed with the temporary stuff of life.

Then, our doctor calls us up and says there's something funny with this X-ray or that blood test, and we suddenly realize how mortal we are, and how dependent we are on God.

Don't forget those wake-up calls.

September 11, 2001, shook up a lot of people in North America. Perhaps for the first time since the Second World War, we realize how vulnerable we all are. If you'd interviewed even just one of the 5,000-plus people who died on that day, none of them would have been expecting it.

As we all watched with horror as those towers imploded, for a moment we identified with those people and their families. We realized it could just as easily have happened to us.

A Chicago businessman was on the 105th-storey of the World Trade Center when the terrorist strike happened. He was fortunate enough to find his way out just before it collapsed. In an interview with the press, he kept saying: "I will never take life for granted again, I will never take life for granted again."

He's been looking at his life differently. He's looking at his faith differently. He's been looking at people differently, and at his family differently.

Remember those wake-up calls in your life. They will help you to understand in a whole new way, what's really going to matter in the end.

In Psalm 90, the psalmist is reflecting upon the brevity of life:

"Lord, you have been our dwelling place throughout all generations. Before the mountains were born, or you brought forth the earth and the world, from everlasting to everlasting, you are God...For a thousand years in your sight are like a day that has just gone by....

The length of our days is seventy years — or eighty, if we have the strength; yet their span is but trouble and sorrow, for they quickly pass, and we fly away...

Teach us to number our days aright, that we may gain a heart of wisdom."

Remembering to number our days makes us face the fact that one day the numbers will run out. It makes us face our mortality. Death can be a teacher of wisdom.

When I was informed that I had cancer, I was stunned when the doctor told me of the news, trying to process the fact that I might die. I remember hugging my wife, just not wanting to let go.

Then, 12 years later, when I had my second bout with cancer, I remember hugging each of my boys and trying to come to grips with the reality that I might not see them grow up. In a matter of hours, my life was turned — not upside-down, but right-side-up.

The Lord enrolled me in his graduate school of suffering, and He began to teach me to number my days aright. I learned what was really important in life. I wanted the kind of life that He wanted me to live — the kind of life that I could rejoice in, the day I closed my eyes for the last time.

This left me with a daily awareness that my very life is in His hands, that every heartbeat is a gift from Him.

Numbering my days changed my relationship with my family. A day didn't pass that I didn't tell each one of them how much I loved them, and why. I was much more patient with them, far more open with them about my fears, cares and concerns, far more quick to say 'I'm sorry.' It's amazing how little pride you actually have, how unimportant it is to win an argument, or be right, when you realize you may be dying.

Remember, this world is not our home — we're just passing through.

My experience in the graduate school of suffering also gave me a special compassion for those facing hardship. 2 Corinthians 1:3 reads "*...the God of all comfort...comforts us in all our troubles, so that we can comfort those in any trouble with the comfort we ourselves have received from God*." Without tears, our eyes would never be cleansed to see the needs of others who are in pain.

When I first heard about a young mother in our church, whose vibrant life had been interrupted by a strange disease that left her physically helpless, my heart went out to her and even though thousands attend our church, I made a point of visiting with Grace in the hospital.

In my first visit, she was at one of her lowest moments. She was hardly able to move and though she put on a brave face, I could sense her confusion and frustration.

She needed encouragement, and so I shared with her a few thoughts on what I had learned through my time in "the valley." I said to her, "When you are in the valley, you can have people all around you and you still feel lonely and fearful and confused. Only God can meet you and minister to you in the valley." In Psalm 23, we read, "*Even though I walk through the valley of the shadow of death, I will fear no evil, for You are with me*."

In the darkest, deepest valleys, I made a decision to put my trust and hope in God and God alone — constantly rehearsing the truth of what the Bible says about Him — that He is faithful, that He can be trusted, that He loves me more than I could love my own children, that He is totally aware of what is going on in my life, and that He has my best interest at heart in all things — regardless of what I may be experiencing at the moment. I hung unto these truths with a pit-bull faith. The result was a peace that passes all human understanding.

Later, I was to learn that my testimony of God's faithfulness served to inspire Grace — and it has been amazing to watch Grace deal with the challenges of her illness with courage, grace, peace and even joy.

Now it is her turn to inspire you. Her story will not only give you greater insight into the trauma and challenges of chronic illness, but will offer comfort, encouragement and hope.

I'm very thirsty.

I can see my water bottle on the bedside table. A nurse must have moved it when I wasn't paying attention.

I always make sure to keep it beside me on the bed, in case I need it. On the table, it's as distant to me as if it were across the street. Or in China.

I am lying on my back, staring at a glowing bit of light creeping onto my ceiling from the hallway — somebody left my door open.

I can barely move. I can't get out of bed to get over to the table. I can't even lift my shoulder or roll over.

The nurses are supposed to turn me every two hours during the night, to avoid bedsores. But they hardly ever do it.

My mouth is so dry. I think I'm running a fever.

My arms are so weak and stiff; I can't reach over to press the "call" button to get help from a nurse. To compensate, they've set me up with a mobile call unit that can be placed right beside my hand. But the last nurse moved it and forgot to put it back on the bed.

I try calling for help, but nobody seems to hear me.

I feel totally alone. Sleepless, I stare at the ceiling.

What is happening to me?

Am I dying?

Is this my life now? What kind of life is this?

I'm all alone. Does anyone care?

Oh God, please help me.

Chapter One

WHY ME, GOD?

"Praise the Lord, O my soul; all my inmost being; praise his holy name. Praise the Lord, O my soul, and forget not all his benefits — who forgives all your sins and heals all your diseases, who redeems your life from the pit and crowns you with love and compassion, who satisfies your desires with good things so that your youth is renewed like the eagle's."

Psalm 103:1-5

There are no guarantees in life.

We all know it.

We nod our heads sagely to such idioms as: "Live one day at a time" or "Nobody knows what tomorrow will bring."

Those platitudes seem fairly obvious, but they're also very true.

Regardless of our age, gender, education or socio-economic status— illness or accidents can strike anyone at any time.

In fact, one can be happily living one's life, enjoying a new baby, a devoted spouse and an interesting career and then, in almost no time at all, be confined to a wheelchair, unable to even roll over or feed one's self.

I know, because it happened to me.

In my darkest days and weeks of illness, I was considered to be almost a quadriplegic, unable to accomplish even the simplest tasks.

I can't fully convey my sense of absolute dismay and humiliation when I got to the point that even matters of personal hygiene and using the washroom required significant assistance, first from family members, and then from strangers.

But as bad as the physical aspects of chronic illness can be — and they can be terrible — they almost pale compared to the psychological torments we can go through. Uncertainty, despair and fear constantly attack the ill and their families, despite any amount of pep talks or forced optimism.

Chronically ill people may worry about dying or future sufferings. They wonder if they'll ever recover sufficiently to lead a "normal" life. They worry about whether their loved ones are coping, and may even fear abandonment.

Every one of us will eventually face death. However, healthy people may not necessarily think about that fact very often. But the chronically ill person is much more aware of the frailties and treacheries of these human bodies.

People with chronic illness have a condition that they'll probably have to deal with throughout their lives. So the real issue isn't about dying; it's about *living* — and doing that in a way that's effective and rewarding, regardless of the illness.

People with chronic illness come to understand that there are no guarantees for anyone. All any of us have for certain is today; so we need to make the most of it!

Some patients and commentators even advocate "embracing" the illness, as one becomes so much more appreciative of the health we do have, and the good days.

Personally, I'm not ever sure I'll be happy to have Lupus, but I will admit it's forced me to focus on what's truly important in my life, and that's a good thing!

Nonetheless, being diagnosed with a disease of any sort is undeniably traumatic.

A lot of so-called experts have tried to outline and classify the "stages of grief" that a person goes through when they're diagnosed with a serious illness. A quick search on the Internet, for instance, will quickly produce documents on "*The Five Stages of Grief*," the "*Seven Stages of Grief*" and the "*Ten Stages of Grief*." The real point is not so much how many stages there actually are; but that grieving is a process.

Elizabeth Kubler-Ross may be one of the best-known writers in this area, with her 1969 book, "*On Death and Dying*." In that, she outlined five key stages, including: denial, anger, bargaining, depression and acceptance.

I've never wanted anybody else to tell me how I'm supposed to feel. Nonetheless, the chronically ill person can probably expect to go through all the above emotions at some point. In fact, some people might experience a few of those responses at once, and regularly alternate back and forth between them. And despite everything, even the most emotionally healthy person who is faced with serious illness will at least occasionally feel depressed or even angry — and that's a very normal response!

In "*From the Ashes of My Dreams*," Ed Smith writes about his own response to the accident that left him a quadriplegic — and his questions of God. *"And then this happens. Why? People keep telling me it's all part of a plan, your plan, I assume. But tell me. What grand purpose is served by me being in a wheelchair for the rest of my life? Do you really plan this sort of thing? I'm told you love me. You would do this to someone you love?"*[1]

I've found that to survive — physically and mentally — a person needs to know where his or her centre is. For me, that centre is found in my faith and hope in God to protect, guide and direct my life, even through these unpleasant paths.

I don't know why I was struck with such a serious sickness.

Was God trying to get my attention? If so, knocking me off my feet (literally) might have been a good way to do it. Or, was I being punished for some past sin? Was I not sufficiently thankful for all that I'd been given in life?

It's very easy to get drawn into debates over "Why does God allow bad things to happen to people He loves?" But I do believe that we as humans need to take more responsibility in that discussion. Not only are we stewards of the Earth ("*So God created man in His own image, in the image of God He created him; male and female, he created them.*" Genesis 1:26, NIV), we are creatures with free will and choice. Because of our own errors and weaknesses — and those of our ancestors — we live in an imperfect world, full of suffering, sickness, disease and even death.

In this world, we'll all have to deal with some of these issues.

However, the good news — the great news — is that we don't have to do it alone. Instead, to those who search, they'll find that God is ready, willing and able to provide more than sufficient comfort, guidance and help on the journey.

I don't really adhere to the "everything works together for good" philosophy that we hear about now and then. How can it, when there's obviously so much evil and suffering in the world?

However, what Romans 8:28 actually says, is: "*And we know that in all things God works for the good of those who love him, who have been called according to his purpose.*" That means, if you love God — He is actively working for your good! To take that further, I believe it's not so important to understand *why* bad circumstances happen, as it is to see that there are opportunities for good in *any* circumstance!

For me, such "opportunities for good" have included the development and deepening of my faith, as well as the chance to really focus in on truly important matters — like my family.

When you're seriously ill, it's amazing how trivial so many previously important matters become. If you can't reach your own face, you can't get too excited over who wins the hockey game or even whether or not your child refuses to eat carrots. So serious illness is a wonderful way to concentrate the mind on what's most important!

Moreover, my ability to empathize with sick and disabled people has grown exponentially. I understand too well what it's like to be confined to a wheelchair and a bed. I know what it's like to live in an "institution," to feel that you're no longer viewed as a real person, with the rights and freedoms that entails. And I know firsthand how hard it is to battle the hopelessness that's so often associated with chronic illness.

Why would I want such knowledge? Well, of course if I had the choice, I would rather never be ill or experience any suffering at all.

But the reality of life is that I don't have that choice. And if I'm able to use what I've experienced to better interact with and comfort other people; that's a huge benefit that will serve me well throughout whatever paths the rest of my life will take.

To my surprise, my illness has also given many others around me their own "opportunities for good."

I was humbled and grateful for so many practical expressions of love and goodwill, as so many people gave so much of their time and effort to support my family with prepared meals, baked goods and even babysitting.

Moreover, I know for a fact that literally hundreds of people were diligently praying on my behalf, even when I was too weak and sick to really pray myself. Later, family members confided that they felt their own prayer lives and faith were actually strengthened through that experience.

Despite the best support systems that may be available — from family, friends and health professionals — a person with chronic illness will find that very often, the journey seems a lonely, unique one. While obviously many others have experienced sickness and suffering, their circumstances will never be exactly the same as what you're going through.

For awhile, I found myself responding oddly to hearing other people's stories. In some cases, their problems sounded very trivial to me. Visitors would try to encourage me by telling me how physiotherapy helped their stiff elbow or ankle, while I was struggling to regain the use of almost every muscle in my body. Because their experiences were relatively mild, I couldn't take any comfort from that, and even felt I was being patronized.

Yet when I encountered people with very serious illness who were worse off than me, I often found that depressing and scary — and I'd start to worry if even more dire things could be coming my way.

When I heard of people with my disease who were living normal lives, I admit to feeling not only jealous, but also feeling that they couldn't really understand my predicament, because they hadn't experienced what I'd been through.

Still, I often find it very encouraging to hear about how other people have experienced very serious bouts of illness, and have survived and even triumphed over their disease. Finding someone who's faced something similar to what you're dealing with can be a tremendous source of strength, comfort and encouragement.

I'm choosing to share my own story, not so much because I expect others to find it incredibly special or inspiring, but because it's possible that someone else will find something to relate to, in what happened to me.

When I was gearing up to write this book, I mentioned to my Dad that I was finding it hard to start telling my story, because I don't know how it will end. But he wisely reminded me how none of us really know how our stories will go. And that's okay too, because it's the day-by-day journey that really matters after all!

"*But those who hope in the Lord will renew their strength. They will soar on wings like eagles; they will run and not grow weary, they will walk and not be faint.*"

Isaiah 40:31

Chapter Two

THE BEFORE-TIME

I'm a minister's daughter — a "PK," for "preacher's kid."

In fact, both my parents are ordained ministers. Growing up, they moved me and my two younger sisters, Ruth and Sara, around every few years as they were pastors in a variety of churches in Eastern and Northern Ontario, everywhere from such booming metropolises as Enterprise, Sharbot Lake, South Porcupine and Espanola.

As a PK, it was difficult to change schools every few years, to always be the new kid, especially as I got older.

Moreover, in those small communities, eyes were always on me, to see what the minister's kid was up to. I was supposed to be an example, something my parents reminded me of, and that I deeply resented.

Nonetheless, being constantly exposed to new situations gave me coping skills that would help me in later life. And my parents did their utmost to encourage my interests and development, supporting me through piano and art lessons, public speaking competitions, French immersions and almost everything else I set out to accomplish.

When I turned 18, I headed off to study journalism at Carleton University. It was exciting to be on my own and finally able to make my own decisions; not that I always made the right ones! Thank God for his protection during those years.

In my final year of school, I met a young man studying civil engineering named Douglas VanderVelde. He was tall and lanky with longish blond hair and an on-again, off-again beard. He tended to wear ripped jeans and cowboy boots and I thought he was absolutely wonderful.

We dated for eight months, and Doug proposed shortly after my graduation from university, on a beautiful moonlight night in a small park close to where I was living in Ottawa. We were married about eight months later.

Wedding Woes

Oddly enough, I can't reminisce about my wedding day without thinking about tears and food. More specifically, an excess of crying on all fronts, and to my chagrin — my sudden, inexplicably enormous appetite.

Right up front, let me assure you: I typically eat no more than an average amount of food. Perhaps less! And I'm not a big crier. If you hurt my feelings or step on my toe, I'm generally rather stoic. It's just the touching things that particularly get me. Okay, I blush here, and admit that I'm easily "touched." Alright, alright — I've cried at commercials! But I assure you, only at those extremely heart-wrenching, tear-jerking, touching commercials!

And what could be more touching than one's own wedding day?!

In hindsight, in light of my particular affliction — perhaps I shouldn't have asked my father, conveniently a minister, to perform the ceremony. But really. Should I have known that my dear Dad solemnly uttering the vows with just a slightly sentimentally wistful tone to his voice, would turn on my faucets?

Or could I have known that my two younger sisters, Ruth and Sara, who'd kindly agreed to serve as bridesmaids, would follow my tearful lead? It really wasn't so bad when our backs were to the audience. But when my dear and talented sister Ruth stepped onto stage for her solo, and her song was punctuated by a few well-placed sobs, well — we were all done in for. My parents' congregation was out in full force to witness this oh-so-meaningful event in the life of their minister's eldest daughter, and suddenly, the tears were free-flowing!

I took the opportunity to awkwardly mime at my father until he clued in and smoothly, with the ease of a well-versed professional, slipped me the hanky he carries in his pocket, for emergencies. (If you watch closely, you can catch the memorable moment on the wedding video.)

As we slipped out of the sanctuary and into a receiving line, sobbing ladies gripped me in tight hugs, squeezing out yet more tears. Between them, my father and new husband efficiently set up an almost production-line-like system, to discreetly hand me tissues and whisk away the used rejects.

For years after, my in-laws delighted in rewatching the wedding video, gleefully pointing out each stashing of Kleenex or swipe of a tear-stained cheek.

By the reception, I'd very nearly got the tears under control.

Suddenly, I realized I was utterly ravenous. Soon I had a heaping plate of food in front of me. Then, I had another one.

Oddly, my beloved spouse barely ate a bite of his dinner. Boy, I really coveted those morsels of nourishment!

After the dinner, the speeches and the socializing, our best man whisked us off to the airport, for a short flight to Toronto before heading off the next day on a tropical honeymoon. I couldn't wait until the steward brought around that little plate of sandwiches and fruit. Starving, I quickly ate it up. Then I ate my spouse's.

Finally, we were at our hotel. The bags were stashed away. The door was locked. I was alone with my brand new husband.

He smiled lovingly at me and came closer.

I stared deeply into his big blue eyes, and whispered: "Can we order room service?"

Once upon a time, I had hoped to work on Parliament Hill and cover major political stories, hobnobbing with politicians and other major newsmakers.

But when I graduated in 1991, in the middle of a recession, the only publication that offered me a job was an obscure Toronto newspaper called *Computer Dealer News*. Down to my last $200, I took the job, and left Ottawa for Toronto. Doug obligingly continued his schooling in Toronto to join me, as I launched my career as a technology and business journalist.

A few years later, a competing publishing company hired me away, as an editor, and I worked on various publications there, eventually as Editor of *Computerworld Canada*.

Even though this line of journalism hadn't been my original choice, I found the details of emerging technologies to be quite fascinating.

Plus, the lifestyle was quite fast-paced, as I flew off to press announcements and conferences across Canada, the United States and even Europe. While most of my time was spent in boardrooms or convention centres, I nonetheless had the opportunity to see a bit of many interesting cities and monuments — from the Arc de Triomphe, to the Eiffel Tower, the Coliseum, the Golden Gate Bridge, to the Empire State Building. I even dined in the World Trade Center — a sobering thought when one considers the eventual devastation to hit that structure.

But five years after we arrived in Toronto, we moved all the way across the country so Doug could take over the Calgary office of his family business. As Doug had originally followed me to Toronto, it seemed like it was my turn to follow him, as he pursued his career opportunities.

Socially, it was difficult to give up close proximity to our Toronto friends, and to get even farther away from our families. While we came to truly enjoy Calgary and Alberta, the initial move to a new environment was a tough one, especially for me. Doug was much too busy with his new role in the growing family company to spend a whole lot of time missing Toronto.

With the move, I decided to start freelancing, and began using my Toronto writing contacts to secure a variety of contracts and assignments, mainly about technology and Internet matters. Technology issues that had been rather obscure when I joined the business in 1991 were hot topics in the major newspapers in 1996.

And interestingly, the major newspapers were also eager to have "Western" representation and coverage in their publications. I continued to receive invitations to interesting events around the world. The move to Calgary, which had originally seemed a death-blow to my developing career, actually turned out to be quite beneficial, because as a freelancer, I was able to write for a variety of interesting business and technology publications, including *The Globe and Mail*, the *National Post* and the *Calgary Herald*.

The freelance career also allowed me flexibility with my time schedule, and so I was able to pursue some of my other dreams; such as creative writing. With effort, I managed to complete my first novel, aimed at young adults, a coming-of-age-type story called "*A Hole in the Hedge*,"[2] and began the daunting task of marketing that to publishers.

However, the real tragedy in my life at that point was the lack of a child in our lives; even though doctors hadn't been able to find a reason for it. Finally, we started to look into adoption.

In September 2000, after almost nine years of marriage, our precious son Adam arrived in our lives. We adopted him through "open adoption" — which has a wide-ranging definition, from merely knowing the names and some details of all the parties involved to really active contact arrangements.

Adam's birthfather filled out an information form with the adoption agency, providing medical information, but that was it. However, we had quite regular contact and visits with his birthmother.

A lot of people are quite surprised and concerned when they hear about open adoption. However, the idea behind it is that it's easier on the child to grow up without the questions that inevitably plague many adopted children. They grow up with an awareness of their biological connections and when the time for the "tough questions" arrives; well, they can just pick up the phone. There's no great mystery attached to their existence.

While the concept is lovely, and indeed one that I mainly agree with, I found it sometimes difficult in practice. To my surprise, I initially greatly mourned the lack of a biological connection to my son. And I think the very regular contact with the birthmother, especially in the early days, reinforced that insecurity. I adamantly felt that Adam was my son, but paradoxically, I didn't always feel like I was really his mother.

More than that, I was deeply aware of the birthmother's own pain during some visits, and her reluctance to leave Adam when she visited was obvious. So while the visits generally went well, there seemed to be an undercurrent of sadness that I found quite difficult.

Chapter Three

THE BIRTH OF ADAM

The doctor shouts.

There's a sudden flurry of activity.
He has a baby in his hands.
No wait, he thrusts it on top of her stomach.

Time stops.
There's a child here, right in front of me.
(Why am I so surprised to see an actual child?)
Yes, he's a boy. His big dark eyes look around.
At me.
He's moving his arms and legs.
He has 10 fingers and 10 toes; they're wrinkled and greyish, like tiny elephant limbs.
Yes, 10 fingers and 10 toes.

"Who's cutting the cord?" the doctor barks, hurriedly.

"She is," responds the young woman's mother, pointing at me.

I blink. What?

Someone shoves a pair of gold-toned scissors in my hands.

What?!

Panicked: "I don't know what to do."

The doctor holds the cord. "Just cut between here and here," he says, quietly.

There's a crowd of people gathered around, impatient. I swallow.

My hands move the scissors to the three intertwined veins, and start to cut them. They're tough, hard to get through. Blood drops out of the veins as I cut, flowing over the scissors.

There's still half a vein to go. I glance at the doctor. Did he tell me to keep cutting? Or did I just imagine that?

I cut again.

The room erupts into action, and everyone rushes about. The baby disappears.

No wait, the nurses have him, under a heat lamp, fussing about, cleaning him...

I hold the scissors.
I'd really like to put them down, but they're covered in blood.

I hold them.

Finally, a nurse isn't rushing by.

"Please, may I give these to you?"

Almost everyone is over near the baby, cooing at him. He stares with his big blue eyes.

I am oddly astonished. There's an actual baby here.

Will I really get to take him home?
How could that be?
Or, am I just here, as a witness to this whole amazing process?

Look, look. A real baby's over there.

I stay by the bed and hold her hand.
"He's beautiful," I say.

Her mother hands the baby to my spouse, Doug.

"Can he see?"

We all laugh.

"Of course," her mother says. "Stick out your tongue at him."

The baby mimics the action, showing his tongue in reply.

My husband seems astonished.

The baby holds his mouth wide open, like a tiny bird.

That tugs at something inside me. "He's hungry," I insist, worried.

The nurses tell me it's just a reflex.

The young woman in the bed says I should feed him first.

How truly exciting, to hold this very tiny person, to be the first ever to hold a bottle to his mouth and watch him drink.

He's not very good at it; it runs down his cheek, his chin.

This is overwhelming.

Could I possibly be allowed to take this baby home with me?

I hardly sleep. I hate to leave him, even for a few hours.

Now we leave the hotel, to head back to the hospital.

There are a lot of people in the room. The baby needs his diaper changed. Someone tells me to do it.

Everyone watches my awkward effort.

They're calling him Adam, the name I chose before this baby was born.

Actually, I'd picked other names too.
This was the only suggestion that both she and my spouse didn't dislike.
I stopped asking the other relatives for opinions.

The paediatrician examines Adam, and gives the instructions to me.
I listen, awkwardly uncertain, as everyone watches.

Later, they pack the baby into the car seat we'd brought, and we all leave the hospital.

We hug.
Is everyone crying?

Are we leaving?
Is anyone going to stop us?

I sit beside the baby in the back seat.
He's already asleep.

As we drive away, we see the entrance in the distance. She's sitting on the short stone wall, as her mother brings up their car.
We tentatively wave. She waves.

"Can you believe we've actually got a baby here?" I say, as we begin the three-hour drive home.

"It's hard to believe," says Doug.

I borrow his cell phone and call everybody I know.

"What just happened?" she phones, the next day. "Is the world totally different today, or is it just me?"

I tell her it's totally different.

She's crying on the phone.
We talk for a while. Mostly, I listen, and tell her about what the baby's doing.

He likes to be held. He likes to eat. He's not crazy about sleeping for any length of time. He cries a lot.

Later, when we hang up, I hold the baby and cry too.
Will they take away my baby?

Yes, this is my baby.
Why don't I feel like a mother?

Doug's parents are visiting.

They're very excited about this new grandson, They're laden with presents.

No, no, I say silently. Wait.

Finally. The waiting period is over.
It's official, apparently.

Shouldn't I feel like a mother by now?

"To Adam, you are his mother," says Doug.

It's Thanksgiving Monday. We saved the big dinner for today. We are truly thankful.

This child is actually going to stay in our family.
(Isn't he?)

The months pass. Was there life before Adam?

Adam is a fabulous little person.

He observes absolutely everything.
He smiles and laughs.
He has favorite toys.
He sits by himself, and takes steps when I hold his hands.
He squeals with delight when his Daddy comes home from work.

I hear a stirring in the nursery. I quietly open the door.

Adam is looking right at me. "Ma ma," he says.

I walk to the crib, and he lifts his arms, to be picked up.
"Hug," I say, and hold him close.

I kiss him lightly beneath the ear. He laughs and laughs, and squeezes me tightly around the neck.

This is my son.

I am his mother.

Chapter Four

WHEN DISASTER HITS

"Even though I walk through the valley of the shadow of death, I will fear no evil, for you are with me; your rod and your staff, they comfort me."

Psalm 23:4

In many ways, my life was quite enviable. I had a wonderful child, an excellent husband and an interesting career. I had supportive friends and family.

All in all, things were pretty good, right?

And that's when disease struck.

I can actually pinpoint its arrival in my life to a specific day. That's not really because I have a great memory, but rather because we had just flown to Ottawa to visit my husband's family and to celebrate his May 23rd birthday.

The following day, on May 24, 2001, I noticed a very slight stiffness in my fingers and toes. "Isn't that odd?" I thought to myself.

Over the next few days and weeks it got worse.

It's strange the mental processes we go through in such circumstances. For awhile, I was convinced I had reacted to wearing some new nail polish (donned in honor of Doug's birthday dinner) that apparently contained "Teflon." Alarmed, I diligently scrubbed that off, and waited for the finger stiffness to go away.

When it didn't, I began to fear that I had inherited rheumatoid arthritis from my father, who had just been diagnosed a few years earlier. Before his treatment kicked in, that disease was significantly crippling for him. He struggled to climb stairs. The joints in his fingers swelled up and impaired his fine motor skills. Moreover, Dad lost the stamina and energy that had always characterized him.

But thank God, his doctor was able to get him on medications (which were reduced over time), which allowed him to return to his loved activities, such as walking, biking and woodworking. While the disease continues to rob him of some of the stamina he was accustomed to, at the time I write this, he's still able to live quite an active life.

In June, I saw my family doctor, who sent me for blood tests and arranged to follow up with a full physical the next month. The blood work ruled out rheumatoid arthritis, but did show some "indicators" for another autoimmune disease — Lupus.

It's somewhat odd, because at that very first mention of Lupus, I almost felt a sense of recognition, an agreement that "Yes, indeed, I might have Lupus."

But my doctor told me she didn't really didn't think I had Lupus, despite the blood test, because I didn't seem to have any organ involvement.

There's apparently no clear diagnosis for the disease. Instead, doctors (usually rheumatologists) examine a combination of blood tests and physical symptoms to make their diagnosis.

I really didn't know a whole lot about Lupus at the time, except for the catch phrase I'd seen on television ads: "*The disease of 1,000 faces*." Basically, I quickly learned that it's a disease where the body attacks itself — whether that's skin, joints, muscles, kidneys, the heart or even the brain. No two people with Lupus will have the same symptoms, and the disease can roam about and affect different parts of the body at different times, or even go into remission for long periods.

The biggest symptom for most Lupus sufferers is really serious fatigue — to a degree that most healthy people can't even really comprehend.

Once upon a time, Lupus was considered a fatal disease. But today the experts say most people diagnosed today with Lupus now should expect a relatively normal lifespan (unless they're unlucky enough to have a major attack on a key organ or drug complications!). Then again, I've read that most people with Lupus will never be hospitalized or in a wheelchair — and both happened to me within months of my diagnosis!

By July, I was having difficulty climbing stairs or walking long distances. I was becoming very fatigued, but I attributed that to the demands of parenting. I started to think that age 31 was really just too old to start a family! All my friends were quick to assure me that it was normal to be exhausted with a young child, but it seemed to me that my tiredness was something beyond their own experiences.

Plus, something odd was going on with my right hand. I'd wake up in the morning and it would be "frozen" so I couldn't fully open my fingers. After a few hours, it would relax, and I'd gain full use of that hand again. Even that wasn't terribly troublesome, as I'm left handed, and even the bent fingers were able to type away on my computer keyboard.

As well, my ankles and lower legs swelled up terribly, to the extent that I had triple ankles. I went from wearing size seven shoes to size nine, and eventually resorted to wearing large flipflops whenever I had to leave the house.

When I celebrated my 32nd birthday on August 30, 2001, my husband gave us a weekend away at a mountain resort. As much as I appreciated the thought, I felt terribly ill. It was that weekend I finally accepted that there was something seriously wrong with me.

Doug had taken Adam for a walk, and I went back to my room to rest. However, the cleaning staff were working in there, so I felt I had to leave. But I was feeling so tired and ill; I desperately wanted to lie down! Instead, I returned to the lobby to wait.

I found a payphone and called my mother in Montreal.

Through tears, I finally admitted my own recent realization — whatever was going on with me wasn't simply a matter of stiff joints — I was definitely a sick person. Something was terribly wrong.

Lorna Casselman's *reflections* (my Mom)

"September 11, 2001, was such a disaster to the Western World.

It was also the day that Grace told me that looking after her young son was more than she could handle. By her voice, I could tell that she was extremely ill physically.

On that day when Grace finally mentioned that she was struggling just to look after Adam, I became very concerned. Adam was her pride and joy, and her life. For me, Grace's ability to care for Adam had become the final measuring stick of her physical condition. I was surprised that she had not made that statement earlier — but struggle on she did.

With the disaster in the States and its effect on Canada, the airports were closed down. There was no way to get to Calgary to help out. It was perhaps the most difficult and frustrating day of my life.

To me, Grace's doctors seemed oblivious to how ill she really was. They were treating her as if all her symptoms were just in her mind or that she had a bad virus and it would eventually go away. She was so very ill and none of them were listening. That was obvious to me, but then again, I'm her mother.

I felt that Grace's days, without a miracle, were numbered. By the concern showed by the doctors the day after 9/11, I think the doctors became of the same mind.

We began to ask everyone we knew to pray — for Grace and also for Doug and Adam, and, for a doctor who would really listen to her and find the medical help that she so desperately needed. Phone calls went out and e-mails. The church, which we pastor, began to pray fervently for Grace. We thank God for the people in our church. They were such a blessing to us during those long months and stood by us in some very caring ways.

From many years of walking with God and trusting Him with our lives and the lives of our family, Bob and I, individually and together, took Grace before the "Throne of Grace" in prayer and placed her in God's powerful hands. She weighed heavy on our hearts. We knew that if we didn't place her in God's hands, the burden would be more than we could bear."

Over those summer months, my family doctor gave me various arthritis-type medications, but nothing seemed to be very helpful.

While that time was still far from what I refer to as "my darkest hours," it was undeniably frightening. I had a range of odd symptoms, from inexplicable fatigue, to mobility issues and pain, and significant swelling in my ankles and legs, and eventually my wrists. But no one seemed able to tell me definitively why it was happening, and no one seemed able to help me.

I've heard many times that it's not unusual for people to consider it a relief to be actually diagnosed with a chronic illness. On the face of it, that's hard to believe!

It's probably not true in cases where people weren't aware they were sick. However, in my case, there was a small element of relief to getting a diagnosis, because it brought a certain sense of explanation and the possibility of treatment that could help me. (Of course, I didn't know then that things would get a lot worse before they got better, and that the questions and uncertainties were only going to increase!)

In late September, I was finally able to see a rheumatologist, who officially diagnosed me with Lupus. He immediately put me on a high dose of steroids.

Doug and I were rather taken back by the doctor's bluntness: "They'll make you fat and hairy," he said. (Actually, that's not necessarily true; I dropped about 25 pounds in the following months, and in fact, continued to lose weight after that. Plus, the chemotherapy I eventually had took care of any extra "hairiness.")

While I experienced an immediate surge in energy and the reduction of certain symptoms, like ankle swelling, within a couple of weeks my mobility continued to decline very quickly. Soon I had real difficulty with stairs, or even getting up out of chairs.

Ruth Casselman's *reflections* (my sister):

"The news was so potentially devastating that my first reaction was to minimize the emotional impact that it could have on my daily life. I really didn't want to talk about it, or even to think about it at all.

It was like I was a little kid again, and I'd put my hands over my eyes to make the scary things go away.

But, every time the phone would ring, I would be forced to face the fact that my sister was sick. Very sick. And the process of facing reality was painful and heartbreaking, every single time."

I had thought I was having problems with my joints. While that may have been partly a factor, my rheumatologist told me that the disease was actually attacking my muscles. Moreover, more blood work raised the possibility of a kidney issue, so he referred me to a kidney specialist, called a nephrologist.

The nephrologist recommended a kidney biopsy, which was scheduled for early November.

But the day I was supposed to go to the hospital for the biopsy, I awoke with a raging fever that approached 40 Celsius. ("Low grade" fevers are a common symptom associated with Lupus.)

By this point, I needed help to get out of chairs. And in the waiting room, I asked Doug to put his arm around me on the sofa, because I wasn't strong enough to sit upright on my own.

And when I went in to have the biopsy done, I wasn't even able to roll over onto my stomach without help from the medical staff.

As I lay in "recovery" after what should have been just a minor day surgery, the nurses were so distressed by my persistent high fever that they paged my nephrologist, who had me admitted to hospital.

I was given three days worth of high-dose intravenous steroids to try to shock my system out of its attack on my muscles, but there was no noticeable effect. I've heard other people talk about their reactions to such treatments, such as major mood swings. Personally, I didn't notice any significant side effects, but likewise I didn't notice any improvements!

Fortunately, the results of the kidney biopsy showed very little damage. So typically, as my kidneys were relatively healthy, I would have been sent home with occasional doctor visits to monitor the situation. Even though I was lying in a nephrology ward, my biggest problem was obviously to do with my muscles.

The nephrologists, in consultation with hospital rheumatologists and neurologists (brain, nerves and muscle specialists) decided to opt for a fairly drastic treatment — chemotherapy. While the doses of the intravenous drug for Lupus are much less than those given to cancer patients, it's still a fairly horrible experience with all kinds of potential side effects, ranging from nausea to fevers, hair loss, and even the development of various cancers.

I experienced a lot of fatigue for days and even weeks after the chemo treatment, and felt a bit nauseous, although I was spared the vomiting episodes so often associated with chemotherapy. I didn't lose all my hair, but it noticeably thinned out.

In hindsight, I look back at many of my experiences and see them as opportunities for learning, and to empathize with disabled and sick people. But even then, I asked myself — did I really need to learn how to empathize with balding men?

Still, I feel like I can better relate to the various trials faced by cancer patients since I've been through very strenuous medical treatments myself.

Lorna Casselman's *reflections*:

"It was so very difficult to see my daughter now needing help with every part of life.

Her range of movement was confined to a few inches. Water, which she was constantly drinking because of the high fevers, had to be placed in just the right spot or she could not reach it. The nurse's bell was the same.

Grace could still shuffle along slowly if someone would position her to get out of bed and lift her to a standing position. Any movement was extremely painful to her. A nurse told us that a short shuffling slow walk in the hospital corridor had the same effect on Grace's heart that being on a treadmill for many minutes would have on us."

After my first bout of chemotherapy, the doctors decided to send me home — eight days after my arrival for the kidney biopsy day surgery.

My husband carried me up the 28 stairs between my front door and my bedroom, and for the next 10 days I stayed on that top floor and he (and my Mom, who flew out to help) brought me food and visited me in that small space, which consisted of our bedroom, two washrooms, Adam's room and my office.

Believe it or not, I continued to work away on an editing contract I had, even when it became impossible to get off my office chair without assistance.

Doug, with help and advice from the hospital's occupational therapy staff, set up one bathroom with specialized equipment — a raised toilet seat, a special shower bar and a shower seat — but soon even those weren't enough to allow me to cope on my own.

I continued to get worse.

Doug soon had to lift me in and out of beds, and off chairs, and help me wash, and even helped me roll onto my side at night when I got uncomfortable and needed a change of position.

In desperation, he called the nephrologist, who told him to bring me to the emergency department.

After a five-hour wait involving Doug holding me up in a chair, we were finally brought into the emergency department and eventually seen by a neurologist. (While waiting for a room to be available, I spent a certain amount of time lying on a stretcher in the hall, while a half-naked drunk man wandered around me, asking people for a "light." I begged Doug not to leave me, as I lay virtually helpless in the middle of what seemed rather like a TV hospital drama.)

Eventually staff found me a room on the neurology ward. The doctors tried another dose of intravenous steroids. Along with the continued chemotherapy, they also gave me a blood product called gamma gobulin. That involved being hooked up to an IV for four or five hours per day, for five days at a time.

I was dehydrated from regular fevers, so they'd regularly pump saline solution into me. I was also severely anaemic, so at one point the doctors prescribed a five-day intravenous iron treatment. For awhile, it seemed I was almost constantly connected to an IV machine, and my hands and arms started to look (and feel!) like pincushions.

The nurses often seemed to have great difficulty getting the IV needle into my hands and wrists — which I found to be a very painful process compared to getting blood taken, for instance — something else that was a daily occurrence for awhile.

Often they'd insert the needle, just to tell me it was no good, the vein had collapsed. And to make it worse, the hospital has some sort of rule that a nurse is only allowed to try twice, so that after a failure, I'd have to lie there and wait for another nurse to be found. It seemed that only certain nurses were authorized or willing to do this, and the more difficulty they had with me, the further afield the call would go, most often to the cancer ward, where the nurses had considerable experience with inserting IVs. It got to the point that I desperately wanted to interrupt the first nurse attempting the insertion to ask: "Can't you just send for the good nurse right away?" (Only my so-polite Canadian upbringing stopped me from actually saying this.)

Once, it took seven tries. I distinctly remember two nurses hovering over my arm, and three others leaning over the other side of my bed, all commenting on the state of my veins.

Fighting back tears as yet another needle was painfully inserted, and then another vein collapsed, I gasped: "This must be what hell is like."

"No, no," the nurse rebuked me. "Hell is much worse than this."

"Yes," I acknowledged, chastened.

Then I added. "But this is how it starts."

She didn't argue.

Lorna Casselman's *reflections*:

"Within a few days of being home, Grace was back in the hospital. One by one her muscles seized up. She was losing more and more

movement.

There came a time when she could no longer talk on the phone because she could not hold the phone. I sent her my headphone set but she could only use it if someone put it on for her. Our conversations became extremely short, as she had no strength. Her breathing was very labored and she could only talk with great effort.

I became the link between Grace and her sisters. She did not have the energy to talk. Then the day came when she had no energy and we had to depend on Doug and the nurses to let us know what was happening.

Eating became a major challenge, as she could no longer use a regular fork. The hospital staff and Doug were ingenious in coming up with solutions.

But she was so sick that often the solutions quickly became obsolete."

I'm sitting in the wheelchair, at the edge of the hospital lobby. It's a small excursion for me. Doug has gone up the few stairs into the little café to get us a drink and a snack.

People rush past me. I feel like I'm a bit in the way. And yet I feel invisible. No one really looks at me, or makes eye contact. I'm no longer a young woman, I'm a thing in the way.

That was a frightening, frustrating time, as it seemed like the doctors weren't exactly sure how to treat me, so they kept trying additional things, hoping something, somehow, would have some effect. (Likewise, once I did start to improve, the doctors were uncertain which treatment had helped. So just to be sure; they gave most of them to me again!)

But for days and even weeks, my problems seemed to go from bad to worse. Not only did I continue to worsen in the hospital, I began to stiffen from spending so much time in bed. So not only was I incredibly weak, my arms and legs wouldn't totally straighten. I lost flexibility in my hips, ankles, wrists, elbows, fingers and neck. The "proximal" muscles — those nearest to the body, such as upper arms and thighs — were most affected, which was why I lost the necessary strength to get out of chairs, climb stairs or lift my arms enough to reach my face.

I couldn't put food directly in my mouth although I could usually manage with the extra reach of a spoon or fork, and by drinking out of a straw. Even then, I couldn't reach to the back of the hospital tray, so I could only eat what was at the very front of the tray unless someone wandered by who was kind enough to shuffle the food items for me. (Looking back, some of my requests may have seemed odd to hospital staff who didn't know my situation!)

Ruth Casselman's *reflections*:

"What do you say to a loved one who is facing a terrifying disease?

I asked myself this question every time I spoke to Grace while she was in the hospital.

I wanted to tell her that everything was "going to be alright," but I didn't really believe it myself.

Did she want me to be optimistic or supportive or sympathetic? Did she want me to cry with her? Or make her laugh?

Everything about me and my daily life seemed so unimportant and superficial, but maybe she wanted to hear about something going on outside of the hospital, or maybe, hearing about these things, while knowing that she was unable to do them herself, would just depress her.

As much as I wanted to "be there" for Grace, I really didn't know how. With me living in Ontario and her in Alberta, I couldn't be there physically, and emotionally, I was finding it hard just to keep myself together, never mind providing Grace with the emotional support that I didn't even know how to give."

Each morning, a member of the physiotherapy staff would come to my room to "stretch" me — something that Doug had to take over when I was eventually allowed home on the weekends. (He also had to give me needles in the stomach twice a day, until the medical professionals deemed I was moving enough to minimize the danger of blood clots.)

When I wasn't receiving medical treatment, I spent much of my days with the physiotherapists, who stretched me and worked with me to try and regain strength and flexibility.

What agony!

In those first days, it would often take two or three people just to try and stretch me out, or to get me out of the wheelchair to standing.

I dreaded going to physiotherapy, as it seemed a source of immense pain and exhaustion. And yet, I quickly realized that as tiring as the ordeal was, it helped me significantly — particularly in the area of flexibility.

No one is certain what treatments or exercises were most effective in helping me, but one day, instead of worsening, I saw a slight improvement. Indeed, in those early days, the advances were small, but I noticed them, even if it was just regaining a centimetre of flexibility.

But before long I was able to accomplish some simple tasks like reaching the call button on the side of the hospital bed, or even putting my glasses on. With each minor triumph, I would call my Mom, who would faithfully report the good news back to her vast prayer chain.

Although I began to improve, I had no idea what the future would bring, and no one else seemed to know either.

I did seriously ask my doctors if I was dying, and they assured me I wasn't. (However, I believe they honestly didn't know what was going on with me. And if any of them thought I was dying, I'm not sure they would have told me about it anyhow.)

Later, however, many readily admitted to a great deal of alarm over the seriousness of my condition and the speed of my decline. (Likewise, they were surprised and impressed with the speed of the initial phase of my recovery when it finally happened!)

Even on my more optimistic days, it seemed a very strong possibility to me that I would spend my life in a wheelchair. As I worked with the physiotherapists to regain my strength and flexibility, I told myself that if I had to sit in a wheelchair, I wanted, at least, to be able to use my arms and hands adequately. I reasoned that in that case, I could lead a semi-normal life. After all, didn't I see people zipping around in sporty-type wheelchairs, popping up onto curbs and even driving specially equipped vehicles? And I'd be able to type and continue my career with some sort of writing, be it journalism, creative or editing.

The problem was, with very little upper body strength, I could only push myself a very short distance in the wheelchair before I was exhausted. In fact, when the therapists changed the chair I was in, I couldn't even manage to put the brakes on. That was a source of some fear to me, as I envisioned myself uncontrollably rolling away. (That scenario actually wasn't very likely, as I could reach out and grip the wheels to stop them turning.)

I tried to explain my fears to one of my therapists. "This brake is too hard for me to push on," I said. She encouraged me to keep trying.

"But I'm afraid of rolling away down hills," I confided.

"Hills!" she exclaimed. "There are no hills in the hospital!"

"But what about when I leave the hospital?" I asked.

"Why Grace," she exclaimed. "You'll be walking!"

I didn't entirely believe her, but I admit to being somewhat cheered by the optimism.

I really had no idea in those darkest days what to expect.

Of course, no one actually knows what will happen in the future. But the possibility that my existence could be rather grim loomed large, despite the regular encouragement I received from family and friends.

I never doubted God's ability to heal. But likewise, I know there are so many circumstances where, despite fervent prayers, things don't turn out the way we hope. Not everyone gets healed, and not everyone survives serious illness. Despite wistful thinking, it seemed quite possible to me that perhaps it was indeed God's will for my life to be confined to a wheelchair.

Of course, that's not what my mother told me. She was determined to believe that I'd return to health, even when I could barely move. Meanwhile, she herself received a lot of support and encouragement from others, as she'd get so many reports of people praying for me, even waking up in the middle of the night feeling compelled to pray on my behalf.

My mother constantly told me stories of encouragement from all sorts of strangers who were praying diligently for me.

Perveen Khokhar, a Christian psychologist in Montreal, not only lent her prayers, but she reminded my mother that we serve *"...the God who gives life to the dead and calls things that are not as though they were*" (Romans 4:17).

That verse, she told Mom, applied to me. That even though I wasn't healthy, I should be "called to health" in prayer, because that was God's plan for my life.

They've drawn the curtain all around my bed. It's night, but there's a light somewhere, casting an odd glowing on me, through the curtain.

I am all alone, except for God. There is nothing I can do for anyone else, for my family, for my son — I have to leave them to God's care.

And yet, I am profoundly aware of God's presence, and His care for me.

For me, a major psychological shift happened the day the senior minister at our church, Dr. Henry Schorr, came to visit me in the hospital. He shared a bit of his own story about his battle with cancer a few years earlier and how it strengthened his faith and changed his ministry. And he prayed with me.

Somehow, despite the fact that the visit was brief, it sparked something in me. Not only was I able to start to think about some positive opportunities for me that were occurring because of my illness, but I began to have a genuine conviction that I was going to get better, even though my minister hadn't made any such prediction!

Of course I had moments of doubt, and I still do! But overall, even though my improvements were still extremely modest, I really started to believe that I would not spend my life immobile. When my family came to visit, I would try to reassure them: "I'm going to get better."

"Well, of course you are," they'd reply.

"No," I'd insist. "I'm really going to get better."

"Yes, we know," they'd tell me.

Somehow, I found that disappointing, although I think it would have been considerably worse if they'd questioned or argued against my assertion. But I don't think anyone really realized that a significant mental shift had occurred for me. I went from really having no idea what was happening to me, to making a conscious decision to believe I would get better, and that I would work very hard and endure whatever I had to, to do my part to make that happen.

Through my own experiences, my belief in the importance of a positive attitude has grown significantly. I don't think it can be over-emphasized for anyone, but it's particularly crucial for people recovering from serious illness.

My early gains were extremely subtle, perhaps only that I would realize I could reach one hand a centimetre farther.

It was a day of great joy for me when I was able to get off the hospital toilet on my own (a raised unit with a bar for the disabled).

The humiliation of having to have help with such personal tasks was incredibly demoralizing for me. Very few people can completely understand my sense of overwhelming happiness and thankfulness when I accomplished that simple task.

While I still needed help to stand from the bed or most chairs, I started to be able to walk a little farther and was steadier once I was up.

Then, I was moved off the neurology ward, to the physiotherapy/ rehabilitation unit — quite a frightening prospect at first, as medical care was minimal and the focus was specifically on getting the patients back into their lives. For someone with very limited strength, the prospect of being required to do a whole lot more for myself again seemed daunting.

Lorna Casselman's *reflections*:

"I flew out to Calgary for a quick visit before Christmas.

For two days, I trailed Grace, now in a wheelchair, around the hospital to appointments and therapy.

The least movement was a huge challenge. She was trying so hard. The therapists pushed her as hard as they could, looking for one more centimetre of reach.

I will never forget when one of her doctors walked into her room and said, 'Grace, your condition has finally stabilized. We are going to move you to the physiotherapy building.'

That was the first good news that we had heard. I was able to pack her up and then get her settled into her new room before I left. When one is lying in bed, almost immobile, it is difficult to imagine a "move." I felt that the Lord had ordered my steps in letting me be there.

I will also never forget the morning I had to leave.

The nurses on that wing knew I was heading back to Montreal that morning and that I would come to the hospital for an hour before making my way to the airport.

I came, spent a short while with Grace, and then said my goodbyes, making my way to the hall, only to see two nurses standing at the door. One nurse immediately went to Grace who now was crying horrendous sobs. This was so hard for her. She had no idea that she could be heard outside of her room.

The other nurse linked her arm in mine and walked me down that hallway to the elevators (Grace's sobs could be heard all during that long walk).

This nurse talked the whole way saying such things as: 'Mrs. Casselman, you have to get back to Montreal now but your daughter is in good hands... We are going to get her walking and moving about again. You will be surprised at what will happen in the next few days.'

That scene will forever be on my heart. But I realized then that my daughter was in good hands no matter how hard the next few days would be on her. If the nurses were that clued in to what was happening in Grace's life, they would do all they could to help her to become mobile again."

Even getting myself to the dining room on the rehab unit — trays weren't brought to the rooms — was rather scary, as I barely had the strength to push my wheelchair that distance. It soon become apparent to me that walking would be easier, if only I could get the strength to do it.

I was determined to push the envelope, and push it hard. I started to walk as much as possible, even though I felt very weak, and I would never be sure that I'd have enough strength to get back to my room. Plus, because I couldn't get up if I sat down — I didn't have the option of sitting down to rest!

I tried using a walker, and while it had some benefits as something to lean on, it was also something that required pushing about, and so seemed rather inconvenient. Likewise, a cane was something to be carried about, which felt like a waste of my very limited strength.

"Do you need help with your egg?" the nurse asked.

"Hmm," I said, considering the hard-boiled egg lying on my tray. I was getting stronger, perhaps I could manage it.

"I'm not sure," I answered honestly.

"Well, try then," she said.

I picked up my knife and raised it high, bringing it down on the egg with all my force.

BANG!! The knife smacked through the egg onto the plate so hard it shook the whole tray and sound reverberated throughout the room. The other patients paused and stared at me.

"I think I've got it," I said to the nurse.

I laughed so hard that tears were running down my face.

The day arrived when I could stand on my own from my wheelchair — which was higher than most chairs. But once I started walking, I refused to travel in my wheelchair.

However, for awhile I did walk around pushing the chair in front of me, as I went to my meals in the unit's dining room, or down to physio sessions. I was able to sit on it, and then get up again on my own. (The regular dining room chairs were too low for me to get out of without help.)

Pushing the empty chair around did prompt a lot of questions, but it seemed a reasonable solution to achieving more independence.

One of my therapists suggested I just carry the cushion, and put it on other chairs for added height. I tried that for one day. However, the cushion was large and unwieldy and actually fairly heavy to carry about. Plus I was afraid of losing it! As well, walking about hugging a huge cushion looked rather odd too. I joked that people were going to think I was unusually attached to my chair — first pushing it everywhere I went, and then refusing to leave the cushion behind. I said that next I was going to insist on carrying a thread from the chair around with me. (I was kidding!)

I was allowed to go home for a couple of days over Christmas. It was the first time Doug and I had ever spent Christmas on our own, away from our parents. I had bought small gifts for Adam and Doug from the hospital gift shop — a toy train and a china sailboat, respectively. I was so relieved to be able to spend Christmas with Doug and Adam and not in the hospital, but it was a very subdued holiday for all of us.

Hospital journal, January 2002

"I'm doing very well — walking all over, getting in and out of bed and climbing stairs.

Still, it hurts a lot and it's all hard and exhausting.

I feel ready to go home, but I'm scared too, about being able to cope.

I feel like my life is very boring. It's dull dull dull at the hospital. My weekday activities keep me busy — then it's very dull. If I try to express that to Doug, he just tells me about how miserable his life is.

I love to go home on weekends, but it's dull and uneventful there too.

I could invite visitors over, but I still don't feel confident about feeling well enough to endure the visits. I think my confidence has been shaken too.

I find it hard to hear about all the sad stories of everyone here in rehab. It feels like the human condition is so fleeting and miserable.

I do thank God for all He's done for me and the huge progress I've made. Still, I need His strength to continue onward."

The day came when I realized I could get off most chairs. The physiotherapists declared me ready to go home, and the doctors promptly signed me up for another week of onerous medical treatments and intravenous drugs before I was finally released on January 19, 2002 — almost two months in total in the hospital!

Hospital journal, January 16, 2002

"I'm slated to go home Saturday after my treatment finishes. I'm really looking forward to that, of course.

But I know it will have its own challenges.

I miss Adam. I need to be his mother again.

I cannot believe I've been in the hospital since November. That's a big chunk of my life."

Being home again was wonderful in many ways, as I was able to spend more time with my husband and son. However, there were still a lot of physical challenges to overcome, and a certain loneliness to endure from being relatively house-bound. (For the first few months before I resumed driving, I was reliant on others to take me out. I did make use of the local "Handi-Bus" transportation for the disabled to attend my physiotherapy sessions. That sort of service is wonderful for both the permanently and temporarily disabled.)

While I continued to improve, and returned almost immediately to some freelance journalism from my home office, much of my time continued to be taken up by medical appointments and treatments, including monthly chemotherapy. Those were constant reminders that although I had gained so much strength and flexibility, I still had an underlying disease or "chronic illness" to contend with. And I still battled significant fevers almost every morning.

Even today as I write, I thank God for his mercy to me and for every ounce of physical strength allotted to me. I have no guarantees that this thing called Lupus lingering in my body won't "flare" and attack me again. However, I am optimistic, and I put my trust in God, relying on Him for strength, and most of all — hope.

"Some trust in chariots and some in horses, but we trust in the name of the Lord our God.

They are brought to their knees and fall, but we rise up and stand firm."

Psalm 20:7-8

Chapter Five

THE LONG JOURNEY BACK (and forth, and back and forth)

My little son Adam is a huge fan of the *Teletubbies* — those colourful mesmerizing characters designed to fascinate babies and toddlers. One of his Teletubby videos specializes in nursery rhymes, like this one:

"The grand old Duke of York
He had 10,000 men
He marched them up to the top of the hill
And marched them down again
And when they were up, they were up
And when they were down, they were down
And when they were only half-way up
They were neither up nor down."

As the narrator recites the poem, the colourful Teletubbies march up and down the rolling hills in Teletubbyland, and then fall down laughing.

But for me, that little poem is no laughing matter, because it reminds me of the ups and downs of chronic illness.

For weeks and even months after I got out of the hospital, I continued to improve — to gain strength, endurance and flexibility. Along with my regimen of drugs, I attended physiotherapy as an outpatient, where we stretched, reached high and low objects, climbed stairs and eventually even jogged in the hospital halls!

What I couldn't accomplish one week, I'd have mastered by the next. Finally, by early April, the hospital physiotherapists were content to officially "dismiss" me, provided I would continue exercise programs on my own.

I started going for acupuncture sessions, because I'd heard so many stories of people finding it helpful. (Generally most acupuncturists undertake a "treatment" of perhaps ten visits.) And while I didn't initially experience any huge result, I did show improvement over the weeks, but there were many other factors that contributed, including medical treatments and exercise. With no clear results after nine or ten treatments, weighed against the slight pain of the experience, the cost and the time commitment, I decided to let that lapse.

I also tried massage therapy, which was mainly enjoyable (compared to acupuncture anyhow!), although once again I was unconvinced about its effectiveness in helping me in any long-term way. However, after a few visits, and after my comfort with the therapist grew, and her knowledge of my situation increased, I found my sense of flexibility increased, for a least a few days after each visit. Moreover, the massage itself was pleasant, so I decided to stick with that therapy!

I enrolled in a Tai Chi class, which I'd heard was good for stretching, and started to attend another fitness class as well — one aimed at people with arthritis and fibromyalgia. (I figured the instructors there might be a bit gentle on me; the last thing I wanted was some bulked-up instructor yelling at me to go higher or faster!)

But despite my efforts at exercise, the disease continued to plague me, mainly with high fevers, as well as serious fatigue, stiffness and achiness. A long list of other symptoms included itchy disfiguring rashes, swollen hands and sleeplessness. On the days I felt particularly terrible, I'd abandon the concept of exercise. Then I'd feel extremely bad — a paradoxical situation in which I can be too sick to exercise; which in turn makes me feel even sicker.

And one day it hit me — this could be my life. I'd been working so hard, physically and mentally — to come back from the dehabilitating effects of the attack on my muscles. But no matter how much I achieved, I came to realize that I still had a disease that would torture me for the rest of my life — barring divine intervention and mercy.

That wasn't a light realization. At the still relatively youthful age of 32, I began to understand that as a person with Lupus, I could constantly struggle day-to-day with ill health, while waiting for the disease to seriously flare up in another major attack. Would my health situation constantly fluctuate between bad and worse?

It became amazing to me to watch other people run, walk briskly, rollerblade or even manage several children. How could they have so much energy? How could I have so little? Did they realize how lucky they were to be able to go about life without fighting a losing battle with fatigue, fever and pain?

And yet, I continued to hold onto "my verse" from Isaiah 40: 31 *"But those who hope in the Lord will renew their strength. They will soar on wings like eagles; they will run and not grow weary, they will walk and not be faint."*

I wanted to walk without feeling faint; and the idea of running without growing weary sounded wonderful.

On every front, returning to "normal" life was a struggle. For instance, before driving again, I was forced to not only endure several medical tests, but to actually perform driving simulations and retake my road test — a process that took several months. It seemed barriers loomed at every step.

Moreover, the doctors continued to adjust my medication, regularly creating havoc in my body, both from flares in the disease and side-effects to the drugs.

However, I came to realize that every little action I was able to accomplish was the direct result of God's mercy in my life. I clung desperately to the thought that friends and family continued to pray for me. At my low moments, trembling with fever, I'd telephone my father and he'd earnestly pray for me over the phone lines, stressing that we understood that our hope came from God.

Along with as much prayer as possible and the proper medical care, I can't stress enough the importance of exercise. Most people with chronic illness will be quick to concede that a regime of moderate exercise makes a big difference to their sense of overall health.

For me, as hard as it may be to get out and exercise when I'm not feeling well, it makes a huge difference in terms of pain, flexibility and stamina.

But isn't it ironic? The truly unhealthy among us really must live the healthiest lifestyles!

I don't like to think of myself as vain, but I found it horrifying to realize that I was losing my hair in sizeable quantities. I had already cut it to shoulder length, to make it more manageable in my illness. Then I started to pull my hair back into a ponytail to try to hide the "thinning" spots. Certainly I understood that in the big picture, hair is a very minor thing, and yes, there are hats and even wigs to help out the situation. But still, fighting a losing battle to keep one's hair is a difficult thing, especially for a relatively young woman.

Eventually, I had the hair all chopped off, and decided to start again, with at least initially, a short spiky look. Combined with my weight loss, my appearance was substantially different, something that became very obvious every time I encountered an acquaintance — particularly in business — who hadn't seen me in a year or two. "Grace?" they'd question. "Wow, you've lost a lot of weight," I was told bluntly. "I wouldn't have recognized you."

Sometimes I'd just nod and agree; more often I'd take a moment to explain a bit about what had happened to me.

But even to myself, my unplanned-for "new image" was a bit of an adjustment.

I resumed a limited amount of journalistic writing almost immediately after I was released from hospital. Shortly after that, I heard from a publisher that they were interested in publishing *A Hole in the Hedge*.[3]

Even though it appeared the financial returns would be quite modest, my main interest with that "first" book was just to get it published. Moreover, finally finding a publisher helped validate — if not my writing ability — at least the time spent writing. (It takes a lot of time to write a whole book, and for a professional writer, it was psychologically difficult to write without guarantee of publication.) As a journalist, my articles are always commissioned or assigned before I begin.

In any case, finding a publisher for my first book gave me added incentive to continue with my creative writing efforts. And the timing was excellent — finally a small bit of good news!

I thank God for leading me into a profession — writing — that I'm able to do despite my physical difficulties. The ability to continue with a career (even if that's evolving) has been a positive challenge and comfort to me.

In July, I was delighted to hear that some key blood tests reported almost normal results. I was on top of the hill! But only briefly.

Chapter Six

THE SUFFERING FAMILY

"God sets the lonely in families..."
Psalm 68:6

Hospital journal, November 2001

"How awful is it to be the spouse of someone like me? How long can my husband cope with my helplessness and humiliation?"

Ruth Casselman's *reflections*:

"A close friend of mine lost her mother to cancer when she was only eight years old. Her mother was thirty-five at the time.

This terrifies me.

Grace was only 32 when her disease struck her unexpectedly. I really would have liked to believe that it was impossible for a young woman in her early thirties to succumb to a fatal disease — but it happens.

I guess it can happen to anyone, at any age, but it's not supposed to happen to someone that I know; not to someone that I care about!

I never wanted my sister Grace to be a part of a statistic, but approximately one in 600 Canadians have Lupus.[4] *Grace is too special and talented and unique and important to me, to be that one.*

As miserable as it is to have a serious illness, it's also extremely difficult when someone you care about is diagnosed with disease.

Firstmost, it's heartbreaking to watch one you care about suffer and struggle.

But an illness in the family has a huge impact beyond just the health of one person. Other family members will suddenly have to face increased responsibilities, financial pressures and a host of uncertainties and coping challenges.

Whether the sick person is a spouse, child or parent — life can change dramatically for the whole family.

In my husband's case, his coping strategy was all about problem-solving.

If I couldn't get off the toilet, he bought a raised seat. When I couldn't get out of chairs, he tracked down a special armchair that would virtually lift me to my feet. When I couldn't climb onto the bed anymore, he bought me a step. When I lost the ability to go up steps, he built a wooden ramp. That was just for starters, as he procured a variety of marvellous helps, like my "reacher," which let me pick up things from the floor or drag items off my bedside table; or my "sock aid" which helped me put on socks when I couldn't reach my feet.

But that sort of action approach only takes one so far. The day came (quickly) when virtually every aid that my spouse had tracked down ceased to be sufficient to help me cope with life.

Even as I lay in my bed, practically immobile and reliant on others for almost every aspect of my care, I realized that this whole thing couldn't be much fun for Doug either. When I was at home between my two hospital stints, he had serious responsibilities to do with looking after me, including carrying me around the house, washing and feeding me. Then when I was in hospital, he visited frequently, and at least initially assisted me with many elements of my care.

But beyond that, he was suddenly responsible for looking after a baby full-time! Doug had always been willing to pitch in and change a diaper or prepare a bottle, but that's a big difference from being suddenly thrust into the role of primary caregiver, especially for someone as young as Adam — only 14 months when I went into the hospital.

On top of that, he still had to run his company, with responsibilities to his clients and employees.

Looking back — We had already been married almost nine years when Adam arrived in our lives, so on one hand, we'd already had a lot of time to ourselves, to go out to dinner or the ballet, or to travel. On the other hand, we were rather set in our ways and it was certainly an adjustment to be tied to home and the needs and schedule of a baby. Certainly that was an adjustment for both Doug and me, but I shouldered more of it, as Adam's primary caregiver.

As I began to get sick, but before I was diagnosed, I began to ask more of Doug, as I became overwhelmed with fatigue by the time he got home from work. But he likewise had put in a full day, and the last thing he wanted was to be handed a crying baby while his wife went and lay down. "You wanted a baby," he complained one evening, "but now you don't want to look after him."

In fact, it was heartbreaking to have to admit that I wasn't able to fill the role I'd planned and so looked forward to with Adam's arrival. While Adam was unquestionably "my special person," I was also his — he had a very keen sense of attachment to his Mommy.

It was very hard for me when I went into the hospital, not only to be away from Adam, and unable to parent him in the way I'd planned, but to realize others were caring for him and teaching him, and watching him develop on a day-by-day and moment-by-moment basis while I missed out. That was extremely difficult.

Because I could no longer lift Adam, or really look after him, I felt I was a failure as a mother, and my old doubts about whether I was meant to parent a child returned.

Every visit with Adam was bittersweet, because I loved him so much and desperately wanted to see him. But meanwhile, seeing him only reminded me of how much I was missing.

Meanwhile, I also felt I wasn't much of a spouse — first as fatigue and pain made me feel less enjoyable to be around, and then especially as I became utterly dependent on Doug for almost everything.

(Of note, I even felt like I couldn't be much of a friend, as my fatigue and pain made me feel like I was no longer fun or interesting to be around. And as I became more housebound, it seemed unfairly one-sided for friends to always have to come visit me, when I made no effort to reciprocally travel to their homes. And what did I have to talk about, other than my worsening illness — no doubt a rather depressing visit!)

In regards to Adam, there came a time when I had to emotionally "let him go."

Now that comes for all mothers to some degree, whether it's when they return to work after maternity leave, on the first day of kindergarten, or even as they leave for university! But I had planned to make looking after Adam my primary role in life during his early years, (even though I continued to do a reduced amount of journalistic writing from my home office).

Now suddenly, other people were looking after Adam, and while he always seemed glad to see me, he continued to thrive and develop under their care.

Doug set up photos of Adam in my hospital room. While I appreciated the thought, and although they got a lot of attention from visitors and nurses, I avoided looking at them, because they seemed just a painful reminder of all I was missing.

But eventually there came a point too when I was so ill that I wasn't really capable of thinking about or dealing with much beyond mere survival. And although I was happy to see Adam when Doug brought him to the hospital, that was also an exercise in endurance. His shrieking and occasional crying was probably disruptive to other patients, which made us tense.

Even my own tolerance for his loud baby noises seemed to decrease, and I'd find it very hard to be close to him if he was shrieking. Beyond that, holding him or even having him on my bed was incredibly painful, as he'd bounce on me, crawl on me, and slap my already painful skin in an effort to make a fun noise.

In fact, I came to at least partially dread his visits, as my family would put Adam on my bed, and he'd crawl over me, and jump in excitement — something that was extremely painful on my sore muscles. But I felt that I couldn't ask not to have Adam on me, because what sort of mother doesn't want her son to touch her?

And because I was so reliant on Doug, I needed his attention, whether it was to assist me to the washroom, or to talk about the latest news from the doctors. But there was little possibility for discussion with Adam present.

Eventually we kept Adam's visits to every few days in the hospital, as it was really all I could handle. Still, I felt guilty about even that, and felt very distressed when friends would quiz me about how often Doug brought Adam to see me.

However, Adam was in many ways my inspiration throughout my darkest days. I had the strong conviction that my son needed a mother, and so that gave me extra drive towards my recovery effort. I can't overemphasize the importance of that conviction in my life.

"I have to get better because Adam needs me," I told Doug. "I can't die, because Adam needs me."

Doug muttered something in agreement. Still, he refused to acknowledge that my death from this illness had ever been a strong possibility.

Even when I was at my sickest, he never abandoned the position that I was going to recover, at least to some degree. While most of my other relatives (months later) eventually confessed to fear that I had been dying, Doug still refuses to admit any such thing. Whether it was denial or sheer stubbornness, he was adamant that I was going to recover.

By the time my illness hit full force, Doug had assumed the primary caregiver role for Adam. Our families were back in Ontario and Quebec, so we didn't have any family to lean on for assistance with childcare. Of course, a few friends were generous with their time, stepping in to babysit while Doug went to the hospital. And both my Mom and Doug's mother spent several weeks each out in Calgary to help care for Adam while I was in the hospital, which was so appreciated.

But the whole situation was difficult for Doug, particularly as there was so much uncertainty surrounding the future. While the disease had been creeping up on me, it seemed to hit with sudden severity, and I went, within a few weeks, from basically coping with life, to being a bedridden quadriplegic.

Could I recover from that, and to what degree? What about when I came home? Would the house need modifications? Would I need permanent care? And who was going to look after Adam?

Along with the uncertainty of the whole situation, Doug began to be very sensitive to other people's suggestions and queries. Because we didn't know how my health situation would progress, it was difficult to put a lot of plans into place. And yet, a lot of people were asking us a lot of questions about how we were going to cope — from health providers, to friends and family. He started to view offers of assistance or advice as implications that he was unable to care for his family, and so became (at least privately) defensive and even angry at the people who were trying to help us.

Ultimately, after several weeks of help from visiting relatives, we decided to hire a nanny/housekeeper. I say "we" because Doug talked to me a lot about it, and even brought resumes to my hospital room for my input. That was valuable and comforting because it gave me a sense of parental involvement and even control. However, the reality was I was so sick that I could barely read the resumes, nevermind trying to compare educational and experience backgrounds. I had difficulty focusing my eyes to read, something we attributed to my illness in general. Much later, the problem would be diagnosed as a retinal infection.

The nanny, Dinah, worked weekdays and allowed Doug to return to work more or less full-time, although he did have to look after Adam each night and morning, and weekends. For me, it meant more of an adjustment, as Doug's visits were shorter — usually late afternoon, on his way home from work to relieve the nanny.

Eventually having a nanny also meant someone would be on hand when I returned home, to provide any assistance that might be necessary.

I WANT MY MOMMY

They say nothing's harder for a parent than watching your child suffer.

I know it was very difficult for my own mother on her visits to Calgary to see me virtually helpless, struggling to perform even the simplest tasks. Even though she tried to maintain a cheerful face for my benefit, there were times I saw tears in her eyes as she came upon a nurse washing me, or saw me struggle even with lifting a cup, or watched me push unappealing hospital food around my plate, as I had little appetite, and continued to lose weight.

For me, of course, it was distressing to see my Mom cry, partly because it increased my own doubt and fears about my condition, and it reminded how awful the whole situation must look to others.

And yet, having my mother's help, as well as her emotional and spiritual support was invaluable. She prayed with me, and read scriptures to me. And when I confided that I felt too sick to even pray, she told me that was okay, because she and others were praying for me.

I spent a lot of time on the phone with my sisters, my parents and Doug's parents, and the encouragement they all gave me, and their obvious love and care was incredibly meaningful and helpful to me.

And yet, the physical distance between us was a source of great distress to the entire family, as their access to me was limited. I would have liked to have more of the help and comfort they would have provided if we'd lived closer. But even more interestingly, they too suffered when I was so sick, because they weren't able to be with me.

I am so extremely grateful for my mother's willingness to listen (usually during long phone conversations from my hospital bed, and then later, almost every evening from home) to my every complaint, worry and triumph along this difficult journey. At least in hindsight, I realize it must have been wearing at times to spend so much time hearing about the trivialities of my physical problems, but it has been an immense help and encouragement to me to have someone to talk to in detail about what's going on with me.

I was aware that my Mom was desperately sad at being so far away from me when I was so sick, even though she did manage to fly out to be with me and to help with Adam several times when it was most needed. But as a minister, there were a lot of demands on her back in Montreal, and finances were tight when it came to expensive flights. But she never skimped on listening time.

Certainly, I apprise my husband of significant changes in my health (and he quietly observes more than I even realize without being told), but I'm reluctant to present him each evening with a running tally of what hurts and what doesn't. Rather, if I'm strong enough, I often prefer that we talk about other things, like Adam's development, or life in general. I see part of returning to a normal life as not being constantly focused on my own health. But still, it's great to have someone who is generally willing to hear about every ache, rash or concern, when I feel the need to talk.

"For I know the plans I have for you,' declares the Lord, 'plans

to prosper you and not to harm you, plans to give you hope and a future."

Jeremiah 29:11

Chapter Seven

"Therefore do not worry about tomorrow, for tomorrow will worry about itself. Each day has enough trouble of its own."
Matthew 6:34

"I have told you these things, so that in me you may have peace. In this world you will have trouble. But take heart! I have overcome the world."
John 16:33

THE HOSPITAL EXPERIENCE

Being in the hospital is horrible.

Perhaps a brief stint at the maternity ward might be tolerable, but in general, being hospitalized is just no fun at all. That's particularly true for people forced to endure a long-term stay. Consider this description provided by Elizabeth Kubler-Ross in her book *"On Death and Dying."*

"Well, our presumed patient has now reached the emergency room. He will be surrounded by busy nurses, orderlies, interns, residents, a lab technician perhaps who will take some blood, an electrocardiogram technician who takes the cardiogram. He may be moved to X-ray and he will overhear opinions of his condition and discussions and questions to members of the family. He slowly but surely is beginning to be treated like a thing. He is no longer a person.

Decisions are often made without his opinion. If he tries to rebel, he will be sedated and after hours of waiting and wondering if he has the strength, he will be wheeled into the operating room or intensive treatment unit and become an object of great concern and financial investment.

He may cry for rest, peace and dignity, but he will get infusions, transfusions, a heart machine or tracheostomy if necessary. He may want one single person to stop for one single minute so that he can ask one single question — but he will get a dozen people around the clock, all busily preoccupied with his heart rate, pulse, electrocardiogram or pulmonary functions, his secretions or excretions but not with him as a human being."[5]

On the night I was first admitted to hospital, a nurse sat by my bed and took down various bits of information. "When did you last spend a night in the hospital?" she asked.

"Um, when I was born?" I responded.

Little did I know then that I'd spend most of the next two months institutionalized.

I use the word "institutionalized" deliberately, because that was certainly the situation as I saw it. (In my more sarcastic moments, I've exchanged it for "incarcerated" — just to disconcert friends and family.) Certainly the patient gives up control, and is subject to others' wills, when it comes to sleeping, waking, bathing, eating, exercising or medical procedures. (That's especially true when one is physically incapacitated!)

Over my time in the hospital, I met many doctors and nurses who treated me kindly and respectfully. Having said that, I also encountered medical staff, who if they weren't deliberately cruel, were at least indifferent and unhelpful.

Just like in any profession, some people in the medical field don't like their jobs, or just aren't very good at them. Still, it was somehow a shock to me to realize that not every nurse cared if I got better or not, if I was comfortable. Some saw my needs simply as a task, and didn't seem to recognize me as a real person.

Hospital journal, December 2001

"It's amazing to me how fascinating some nurses find the topic of bowel movements. But it's disconcerting (not to mention too much pressure!) to find a nurse waiting outside the door — or worse yet, coming right in — to inquire about one's bowel movement success."

"A kind, encouraging nurse can make such a difference, even if they're poking me with a needle. (My record so far is seven needle pokes in one day.)"

"There is nothing more frightening than needing help in the middle of the night and pushing the call button — and nobody comes."

"It's horrific to watch one's body rapidly fail. If I can't even roll over, get out of bed, go to the washroom, comb my hair. My body has turned me over to utter humiliation."

"My baby is stronger than I am. If he wants a book or something I'm holding, he just takes it from me, even if I'm holding it with all my strength."

"I'm getting worse and worse — am I dying?"

"Why do friends reassure me that they know I'm going to get better? Nobody knows, and it feels patronizing."

"I am amazed by the extreme kindness of family, friends and

especially strangers."

"Am I supposed to be learning something here?"

When I lived on the physiotherapy ward of the hospital, my life was mostly about pain and hard work, as I tried to regain strength and flexibility. On better days, I compared the experience to being in boot camp, because of the rigid schedules, physical demands, and lack of control over my environment, living in an institution. I was so often at the mercy of nurses and physiotherapists, and they weren't always that merciful.

On bad days, I'd say it was like being a prisoner of war, dragged here and there for treatments and tests while regularly being deprived of sleep by nurses doing rounds and by general hospital noise.

Lorna Casselman's re*flections*:

"There is little or no dignity of personhood in a hospital.

When I have been visiting with members of our congregation in hospitals over the years, I have been amazed at the inconsideration of some in the medical staff. Yet others would go out of their way to help. They were a wonderful blessing. They expressed their concern for the patient and their family in beautiful caring ways.

However, when a patient is physically helpless, some members of the medical staff begin to think that mental and emotional abilities are also lost. I sometimes found myself getting provoked at the lack of personal privacy and at least some semblance of dignity. There is no need for some of the indignities suffered by hospital patients. Sad to say, my daughter also went through a number of these experiences.

Parents are there to look after their children. We are supposed to have the answers. One thing our children are not supposed to do is to leave this world before us. Our hearts go out to all those parents who have children who need constant tender loving care and who perhaps have passed from this life before their parents. The emptiness in their hearts must be terrible. This experience has certainly made me more compassionate to others.

When I am out and see a parent with an obviously "ill" child, I do my best to look them right in the eye and at least smile. When I see a child in a wheelchair, my immediate thought is what can I do to help this parent in this present circumstance. The world in general does not take time for the weak and the sick and the needy."

HOW TO SURVIVE A HOSPITAL STAY

There's nothing particularly fun about staying in the hospital. And the longer the stay, the less fun it is.

Patients are not only ill and away from home, they suddenly have to deal with a relatively unfamiliar environment. And medical staff will now control most aspects of life — ranging from treatments, to when and what the patient eats or even when they can take a bath.

However, patients can and should be prepared to play an active role in shaping their own hospital experience. This is important not only for their own sense of well being, but it could even make a difference to their ultimate health.

Here are some guidelines to consider:

LEARN THE SYSTEM

Life gets easier once you start to understand the system. (Unfortunately that can vary, even from unit to unit within one hospital.) Regardless, taking the time to ask questions about how things work can be very useful.

For instance, particular doctors tend to conduct their rounds at specific times, so with a bit of planning you can make sure to cross their paths, if you have questions that need answering.

Even getting help from nurses is easier if you understand their challenges. For instance, they tend to be extremely busy (and not terribly available) during shift changes, when the oncoming nurses are being briefed and prepped for their new shift.

Of note, don't be hesitant to ask for help. And when you do push the "call button" and a nurse doesn't respond, push the button again! Don't assume you're being deliberately ignored. The person who took your call may have got distracted or your nurse may have been on a break or temporarily unavailable, and your request could have fallen through the cracks. It happens all the time; so keep asking for the help you need!

ASK QUESTIONS, DEMAND ANSWERS

If you don't understand your condition or course of treatment, it's your right to have that information.

Of course, be polite and considerate with your requests. Expressing belligerence or anger will only hurt your cause (even though your frustration may be warranted!) But don't be afraid to ask your doctor for a detailed explanation. There's no need to be shy or hesitant. Despite the best intentions of the medical staff, no one has a greater stake in your health than you do.

DON'T GO IT ALONE

You shouldn't have to deal with the often-confusing hospital system on your own, particularly when you're sick.

If possible, recruit family or friends to help you figure out how everything works. That's where the idea of an "advocate" comes in — someone who can make requests for information or service on your behalf.

STAY ON TOP OF YOUR MEDICATION

This is crucial. Don't assume that the medical professionals are infallible in this area. If someone brings you an unfamiliar pill to swallow, ask what it is. Be aware of what you're taking.

Moreover, talk to your doctor about your medication on a regular basis. Every medication has potential side effects, so it's best to take only as much medication as is absolutely necessary. The doctor may be willing to eliminate or reduce certain treatments if you bring the matter to his or her attention.

For many patients, one of the biggest frustrations is a sense of a lack of control — over their condition, and over their environment. But by making the effort to stay involved, patients can regain control, which is ultimately to everyone's benefit.

THE EMOTIONAL BATTLE

In many ways, the turmoil in our minds rivals the challenge of our physical difficulties.

When one is very sick, or having a bad day, it's very easy to yield to despair and fear. The illness can easily become the key focus of life, as we think about the pain, decreased capacity to contribute or even the prospect of premature death.

Mark Horowitz and Marietta Abrams Brill, the authors of "*Living with Lupus*," write: *"Any chronic illness carries an emotional burden.*

Fear, anger and depression are just a few of the feelings suffered...These emotions are natural. They should not be ignored or pushed aside, but should first be accepted, then understood and dealt with."[6]

And in the forward to Linda Noble Topf's "*You Are Not Your Illness,*" Bernie S. Siegel writes: *"We are all wounded, but we are not all victims. If you learn how to use your inner strength and your spiritual resources, you always have choices and be empowered to make changes or find inner peace."*[7]

Topf talks about how chronic illness (MS), forced her to change her own measurement of self-worth.

"I quickly saw that who I really am is someone more than a person who can no longer walk up stairs or who is becoming less and less able to accomplish certain other tasks in the physical world. Who I am is someone who cannot be validated through my old measurements — that is to say, my old perceptions of self-worth based on accomplishment."[8]

I can relate to that! Typically, my own sense of self-worth has been greatly tied up with my professional endeavors. Have my columns and articles appeared in sufficiently prestigious publications? Am I being invited to cover important events? Am I making enough money from the work that I do?

Later, when Adam arrived, his care and the whole idea of "motherhood" also contributed to my sense of self-worth. And certainly, I still feel that the time I've spent caring for Adam is the very best thing I've ever done.

But what happens when one is too sick to work or even look after one's own child? In such a case, it's very easy to feel that one's sense of self-worth is diminished along with the lessened capacity to contribute to the family's care or income.

In my time of extreme sickness, it became vitally important for me to be able to identify "purpose" in my life, and in my sickness.

I also believe that people with chronic illness have to (with God's help!) develop an enormous strength of will. Sometimes it's sheer determination that forces us out of bed, when our bodies are ready to yield to pain, fatigue or fever. And yet, what is the alternative?

I've had a few friends try to compliment me on my commitment to persevere with exercise or writing, for instance. And certainly one hears regularly about the determination and fortitude exhibited by various sick or disabled people. I believe that's true; and yet, what choice is there?

If I don't exercise regularly, I will get stiff and sore. My stamina will decrease, and I'll feel generally sicker. As much as medical treatments may be important in treating my disease, exercise provides a huge benefit.

Yet having said that, I still struggle with not wanting to do it! If I'm feeling stiff or sore or running a fever, the last thing I want to do is to go exercise! (And sometimes I don't!) But I do believe it's almost always better for me to get at least a moderate amount of exercise than to merely stay in bed and think about how sick I feel.

And it's easy to let life get in the way of exercise. For instance, if I've got assignments due, sometimes I let work take priority over going to an exercise class. But as one fitness instructor pointed out: "Work is no substitute for exercise!"

Many experts will attest to the positive psychological effects of exercise in general. For the chronically ill person, there's the added benefit of getting distracted from the sickness! The sheer experience of getting out and being physically active contributes to a sense of "normalcy" and distracts people from concentrating on an illness.

In general, I've found "distracting myself" — whether it's with exercise, visits with friends, or some sort of outing — is quite effective. The fact is, there are certain days when I'm going to feel less well. Whether I lie in bed all day, or go out to lunch with a friend, I'm going to feel pain and fatigue. And yet, if I can muster the strength to do that lunch, not only will it mostly likely at least partly distract me from the physical pain, I get to experience the joy of conversation with a good friend.

SHOW SOME ATTITUDE

Attitude is critical. When I was in the hospital, I remember a kind nurse telling me a story about two people she'd known who'd had a stroke. They'd had a very similar experience, and both were originally in very bad shape. However, one of the women had a very positive attitude and was determined to recover. She worked very hard and eventually returned to live a normal life.

Meanwhile, the other woman just existed in her illness, and she didn't recover; instead she lived out her days in a special care facility.

Now obviously, there could have been other factors involved, not merely the presence or lack of a positive attitude. Still, that story reinforced the need for personal determination to make the most out of life.

And while one hears talk about "accepting" one's illness, I believe a certain fighting spirit is extremely important. I really do attribute much of my "recovery" to a determination to recover.

I remember very clearly forcing myself to walk all the time as soon as I was able to do, even though I had very little strength and many medical professionals preferred to see me sitting safely in a wheelchair. Then they tried to offer me a walker, but I was determined to walk unassisted.

I met a woman named Gail on the physio unit. I remember her sincerely telling me: "You should never try to get up (out of a wheelchair) without a nurse there to help you."

I disagreed. For starters, the nurses' time was limited, and if I had to count on them for my recovery — well, let's just say I wasn't willing to leave it to them!

The fear was that I'd fall. And I did!

I am walking back to my room after breakfast.

The toe of my shoe catches on the floor. My knee buckles — I just can't recover my balance.

I go down, hard.

My knees take the brunt of the force of the fall, then my forehead smacks on the hard linoleum.

A couple, visiting their son, come running to me. "Are you okay?"

"Please, can you help me up?" I gasp. I am desperate to get up before a nurse comes. I am terribly afraid hospital staff will try to stop me from walking, and make me return to the wheelchair, for safety reasons.

I struggle to get up, and these people who are trying to help don't understand that I need assistance to pull myself up again. I'm on my knees, but I can't get all the way up fast enough. And I can't do it without help to pull me to standing.

The nurses arrive, exclaiming, and asking questions. There seems to be a whole crowd around me. I feel panicked. I'm trying to downplay the fall. "I'm fine, I'm fine, I just tripped."

I feel a bitter sense of desperation. I couldn't get up before the nurses arrived. They pull me up, then take my arm, despite my protests, and lead me to my room. One examines the redness on my knee.

I don't tell them I hit my head. I don't tell them my forehead hurts.

"I'm fine," I tell them. "I just tripped. Everybody trips sometimes."

They hook me to a blood pressure unit, and write something in my file.

"It's no big deal," I tell them. "I just tripped."

Later, when I go to physiotherapy, the therapist says: "I heard you fell today."

"I tripped; it was no big deal," I say. "Everybody trips now and then. I don't know why they made a big fuss about it."

"They have to do a report, if someone falls," she says.

I feel very bitter about this.

But no one tries to keep me from walking.

Now, everything does *not* come down to mind over matter. But the right attitude is certainly helpful!

My friend and former neighbour Sharon suffers from a chronic illness of her own. In fact, people with her disease generally have a lower life expectancy. I asked her how she dealt with that, and her response was: "I guess I feel you have to play the hand that you're dealt."

I think that's a wise strategy. Certainly as I watch people my age jog past my window, or effortlessly hoist their children into the air, sometimes I think it's "not fair."

And yet, is it fair that I have a loving husband and a wonderful son? In many aspects of life, I've been more than fortunate! There's no benefit to trying to judge what is "fair." Rather, we need to deal with what we have, and to make the most of each opportunity that's presented.

More than that, I think it's important to deliberately take things "day by day." Practically, of course we have little choice about it — life unfolds one day at a time. However, many of us spend a lot of time and worry focusing on the unknown future. Instead, it's a lot more productive to live in the moment. When I get up, I can think to myself: "*Oh no, what's going to happen to me next? Is the disease going to strike again?*" Or, I can say: "*I feel pretty good today; what useful/meaningful/fun thing can I do to take advantage of this strength*?"

Dr. Miriam Mollering, one of the ministers at the church I attend here in Calgary, has talked about the importance of focusing not on what we've lost; but on what we have. It may sound simplistic, but it's a good point. I've found that it's not particularly helpful to spend too much time thinking about how much better it was to be healthy, or what it was like to have normal flexibility.

While I continue to work to improve my flexibility, and to live as healthy a lifestyle as possible, it's important to take comfort and joy in my current blessings — my family, dear friends, reasonable mobility, and the opportunity to do interesting work, for instance.

I have heard people afflicted with serious illness or disability refer to their challenges as a "gift." Personally, my generosity of spirit doesn't extend quite that far. Nonetheless, I do accept and even advocate the idea that a serious illness can help an individual focus on what's important in life, identify key goals, and experience the kind of personal growth and empathy that only comes from surviving hardship.

In his autobiography called "*Lucky Man*," actor Michael J. Fox writes about his battle with Parkinson's Disease. He notes: "*...this unexpected crisis forced a fundamental life decision: adopt a siege mentality — or embark upon a journey. Whatever it was — courage? acceptance? wisdom? — that finally allowed me to go down the second road (after spending a few disaster years on the first) was unquestionably a gift — and absent this neuro-physiological catastrophe, I would never have opened it, or been so profoundly enriched. That's why I consider myself a lucky man.*"[9]

And from a broader perspective, a person who has suffered is able to provide perspective and comfort to others in a very meaningful way.

To my surprise, other people have told me they've readjusted how they look at their own lives, after hearing about what I've been through. While this wasn't my intention, apparently the struggles of dealing with a colicky baby seem mild after hearing about how challenging it is to suddenly be unable to even feed one's self.

"*Our suffering always benefits others,*" writes Kay Arthur in "*Lord: Give me a Heart for You.*" She goes on to say: "*And what about that person you've been able to comfort, strength, and support because you understand, because you've been in a situation where you knew God in a way you had not known Him before you suffered? Others saw your example of endurance, and they endured. What greater joy could there be, Beloved, than knowing that whatever trial or tragedy you experienced under the hand of your sovereign God was not wasted but used?"*[10]

Chapter Eight

"Hear my prayer, O Lord; let my cry for help come to you. Do not hide your face from me when I am in distress. Turn your ear to me; when I call, answer me quickly."

Psalm 102:1-2

HOW TO BE A PATIENT ADVOCATE

The single most important help to a hospital person may very well be the help and presence of a strong advocate.

Don't be put off by the term "advocate" — it just means somebody who's willing to stand up and ask questions and make sure the patient receives adequate care.

Of course, the majority of doctors and nurses are working very hard on the patient's behalf. Still, many important matters can — and do — regularly fall through the cracks. That's why it's so crucial to have the assistance of a capable advocate.

While everyone in the hospital can benefit from this kind of support, it's particularly true for the most sick and helpless. I feel so badly for those who are extremely aged or incapacitated, without a committed family or friend to fill the role of advocate.

WHO SHOULD BE AN ADVOCATE?

Ideally, a spouse or close family member makes the best patient advocate, because the medical profession is most willing to release confidential medical information to relatives. However, a patient could try to specifically "authorize" a friend to receive such data. And in any case, even a friend can bring particular needs and questions to the attention of medical staff.

JUST BE THERE

Your presence will, of course, be a great support to your friend or family member. However, if you're a regular presence at the hospital, that will actually contribute to the quality of care a patient will receive. If nursing staff is aware of regular visitors to a hospital room, they may be just slightly more apt to provide excellent care — particularly when the advocate is willing to complain if there are problems!

But beware of this trap: nursing staff may start to view you as a regular fixture. Specifically, if you're constantly around, you may find yourself put to work — assisting with feeding, dressing or even bathing the patient. That may be just fine with you, but if it's not, don't hesitate to merely maintain the role of emotional support for the patient.

EDUCATE YOURSELF

Go into your role as advocate with as much information as possible. Research the patient's condition so that you can talk to doctors and nurses from a position of knowledge.

Moreover, find out as much as possible about the workings of the hospital. For instance, many doctors conduct rounds at approximately the same time each day. By checking with the nursing desk, you may be able to find out when you have the best chance of crossing their path. If you're particularly lucky, the nurse will let the doctor know you'd like a few moments of their time.

TALK TO THE RIGHT PERSON

In some cases, only one specific doctor will be able to answer your questions. In other cases, it will be a particular nurse — perhaps the nurse assigned to the patient on that given day. (Unfortunately that can change on a daily basis.)

It often makes sense to try to talk to the head nurse on any particular hospital unit, often referred to as the "duty nurse." Theoretically this person will have an overall understanding of the entire ward, and is perhaps best positioned to at least direct your queries to the most appropriate people.

BE BOLD

Unfortunately there's a lot of truth to the adage about the squeaky wheel getting grease. Being too timid or easily taking no for an answer won't be of much help to the patient you're trying to assist.

Always be extremely polite but firm when making queries, whether you're asking for re-evaluation of certain medication, or just trying to get the bed changed.

TRY, TRY AGAIN

If your query is important or the patient really needs help with a certain matter, don't give up too easily. Perseverance pays off. Moreover, it's surprising how something may be apparently impossible one day, while it's no big deal the next. That could be merely a matter of a change of staff. If an eager helpful nurse replaces a belligerent one — it can make all the difference in the world. So keep asking!

LISTEN

Paul J. Donahue and Mary E. Siegel, in *"Sick and Tired of Feeling Sick and Tired,"* write: "*Just being a good friend who's willing to listen can't be over-rated. Listening with understanding is an act of love. But it is also a skill that can be learned. In order to learn the skill, you need to identify your non-listening behaviors, that is, all the ways that you respond that do no convey understanding. Then you need to acquire the skill of listening and to practice, practice, practice.*"

Remember, your efforts can make a huge difference to the comfort and even the quick recovery of your friend or family member. So persevere!

HOSPITAL DIPLOMACY

HOW TO PRUDENTLY VISIT A SICK FRIEND

Paying a visit to a sick friend in the hospital is an admirable and hopefully rewarding use of your valuable time. However, certain visits can actually be unnecessarily taxing on the patient's health or good spirits.

At my sickest, I actually didn't want visits — except to see my closest family and my pastor. I felt it took all of my energy just to survive, and I didn't feel I could pull it together well enough to make small talk with visitors. Plus, my quick physical decline was a serious shock for visitors, and I didn't feel I had the emotional strength to see friends reacting to what had happened to me. During those worst times, I actually begged Doug to keep visitors away from me.

While that reaction may seem a bit strange, keeping visitors to a minimum was what I needed at the time. Potential visitors need to be sensitive to the patient's individual situation.

It's important to pay attention to a few simple guidelines when you pay a visit to the hospital.

CALL AHEAD

Surprises are theoretically wonderful, but not always for the hospital patient. If you're not very close family (and even if you are), the patient would probably prefer to know you're on your way.

If the patient doesn't have a phone in their room, check with their unit desk as to visiting hours, and more specifically the patient's schedule. Believe me, they'll appreciate it if you don't arrive in the middle of a sponge bath, for instance. As well, if your friend shares a room, that roommate's habits and schedule could affect the ideal timing of a visit.

If you must show up unexpectedly, consider asking someone at the nurse's station to announce your arrival before marching into the patient's room. That hospital room essentially becomes the patient's bedroom. Even though one comes to accept the unavoidable reality that a certain amount of uninvited medical staff will traipse through at any time of the day or night, that latitude shouldn't have to extend to members of the general public. How would you feel if your casual acquaintances or colleagues suddenly appeared in your bedroom, particularly if you were napping, feeling ill, in the middle of bathing or just being generally dishevelled?

BE ON TIME

It may seem that people in the hospital are just lying around waiting for visitors, but that's not always the case. In fact, many patients are hardly ever in their rooms, and are instead constantly wheeling between tests and treatments throughout the hospital. So don't be surprised if your friend isn't even available — especially if you arrive late or unexpectedly!

When I was in the hospital I had to prepare carefully for visitors. I had such little energy that I liked to take a nap before their arrival. Then I'd call the nurse to help me out of bed so I could primp a little and be sitting in a wheelchair to greet my visitors. However, because I lacked energy, if they were too late arriving, I'd already be extremely tired and fatigued when they walked through the door!

It was a source of serious distress for me that most visitors couldn't seem to understand this. It's just common courtesy: If you say you'll arrive at a certain time, do your best to keep to your word.

BE CAREFUL WHAT YOU SAY

It's quite amazing how hospital visitors can inadvertently be rather insensitive. But there's nothing more disconcerting than having a guest arrive just to blurt out: "Oh, you look terrible!" Or worse yet, is when they immediately start crying at the sight of the patient!

Don't tell horror stories. Everybody knows somebody (or knows somebody who knows someone else) who had a similar disease/ accident — often with terrifying results. Try to refrain from sharing such tales. Even with more positive outcomes, patients still might not want to hear about it.

My initial reactions to such medical stories ranged all over the map, as the months passed. When I was first diagnosed with Lupus, I wanted to know that my friends and family understood this was a significant thing — this was a serious disease that could do very bad things to me, and could, if I was particularly unfortunate, even kill me. So it was distressing for me when people (apparently trying to comfort me), dismissed the disease, or seemed to take it very lightly. "Oh, I know someone with Lupus," they'd say. "She's perfectly fine. It's no big deal."

(Even in those cases where people with serious chronic illness are able to cope with their lives, I question whether casual acquaintances would always know the extent of the struggles and challenges they may go through behind the scenes.)

However, later, as I fought to come back from the horrible attack on my body, I really wanted to hear about other people who'd had extreme physical and health challenges, and who were able to recover from that. Instead, as I moved on in my recovery, it seemed people were suddenly wanting to tell me sad stories. "Oh yes," one gentleman told me. "I knew six people who died of Lupus."

What a strange and disheartening thing to tell someone struggling to be optimistic through a challenging recovery process! (Moreover, I questioned the assertion anyhow — how many people know six Lupus sufferers, nevermind six who died, when the disease is only occasionally fatal?)

As well, please note that this may not be the time to share all your own physical complaints. If you believe sharing your own current or past experiences will be genuinely comforting or inspirational, by all means go ahead. But overall, be sensitive to what the patient may be ready to listen to at this time.

During my hospital stay, I found one visitor quite alarming, as she'd arrive, and then proceed to regale me with her own health woes. While later I came to develop a real interest in hearing about the trials and treatments of all sorts of chronically ill people, at the time I didn't have a lot of patience for what seemed like minor complaints, compared to being almost totally physically incapacitated.

Likewise, I had little sympathy for visitors who would come in ranting about such problems as home redecorating, or trouble with painters. “THIS is your big problem in life?!” I’d silently ask them.

But excess pity or falsely bright optimism aren’t helpful either. Be empathetic, but take your lead from the patient as to what they’d like to talk about. They may or may not want to talk a lot about their medical condition. And that can vary from one visit to another — at one point, the patient may really want to talk about their health struggles. On other occasion, they may be looking for distraction from that, and hope for the chance to talk about other matters.

Be prepared to talk a bit about what’s going on in your life and the outside world — patients can feel very isolated, especially if their hospital stay is a long one.

BRING A THOUGHTFUL GIFT

Of course it’s not necessary to bring a gift at all. However, if you decide to bring something, there may be a few factors to consider. It could be worthwhile to check with a family member or nurse as to whether there are any diet concerns to be aware of. Are there plant allergies? Or is there any counter space available in the room to hold flowers? (There isn’t always!)

And note, something small like a chocolate bar or bottle of juice could be extremely appreciated, especially if the patient isn’t mobile enough to visit the gift shop. Hospital food can quickly become extremely unappetizing!

DON’T STAY TOO LONG

That seems simple enough, but it’s easy to settle in, and most patients won’t ask you to leave. Keep your visit short, especially if your friend’s condition makes them prone to fatigue.

It’s hard to understand the challenges of being a hospital patient, unless you've been unfortunate enough to experience it directly. Nonetheless, by showing just a little extra consideration, your visit will no doubt be highly beneficial to your friend's well being.

Chapter Nine

"...I am the Lord who heals you."
Exodus 15:26

"And the power of the Lord was present for him to heal the sick."
Luke 5:17

WHY DIDN'T GOD HEAL ME? (Or Did He?)

With enormous gratitude I acknowledge and thank the many people who've prayed for me during my time of serious illness and my subsequent battle to recover.

Many of those people possess enormous faith and perseverance, and spent a huge amount of time and effort interceding with the Creator of the Universe on my behalf. I heard stories of various people waking up in the middle of the night, feeling compelled to pray for me. How wonderful and how humbling!

Shortly after my diagnosis, I followed the Biblical principle of going to the elders of the church and asking them to pray for me, which they did diligently. And certainly a number of staunch Christians prayed directly for me at my bedside. That's very Biblical! Take a look at James 5:15 — "*And the prayer offered in faith will make the sick person well; the Lord will raise him up...*"

But with such a backdrop of prayer and faith, why didn't I just leap out of my wheelchair, totally healed? What a great testimony opportunity that would have been! So why didn't it happen?

The short answer is: I don't know!

However, that wasn't God's plan for me, even though I do believe God can and does allow some people to experience miraculous healings, even today. As far as "testimony" potential, the Bible documents many examples of people being healed, and even raised from the dead!

But as my mother reminds me, all healing ultimately comes from God, and I thank Him for the gains I've made, and for every bit of strength I have.

In the well-known book *Joni*, Joni Eareckson, who became a quadriplegic as a result of an accident, writes about two joys. "*One is having God answer all your prayers; the other is not receiving the answer to all your prayers. I believe this because I have found that God knows my needs infinitely better than I know them. And He is utterly dependable, no matter which direction our circumstances take us.*"[12]

For me, my recovery felt painstakingly slow, as I regained flexibility a centimetre at a time, very gradually building up my strength and stamina over many weeks and months. It involved a serious medical and drug regime, as well as significant physical effort on my part, with the help of my physiotherapists.

And yet, more importantly than all those other admittedly helpful factors, I truly believe that God's grace and mercy has been of utmost significance to my recovery process. Moreover, I feel that it was only because of the awareness of God's love and presence that I was able to psychologically and emotionally survive against the waves of fear and despair that surrounded me.

At one point, I even suspected that there must be an angel or two looking out for me. After all, Psalm 91:11 says: "*For he will command his angels concerning you to guard you in all your ways.*"

It started when a hospital social worker appeared at the door to my room and told me my nurse had asked her to stop by.

"My nurse?" I asked, because I didn't have one regular nurse, they changed with their daily shifts.

"Yes, your nurse," she replied.

"Hmm," I said. "What did she look like?"

The young woman stared blankly at me, and I let the point go. But it turned out this person was able to help me significantly to get some information I needed, help with some administrative stuff, and to put me in contact with Lupus support people.

Meanwhile, other small conditions continued to improve, even when I didn't mention them. For instance, someone appeared with a humidifier for my room, which I greatly appreciated, as I found breathing in the dry hospital a challenge. "A nurse told me to bring this," she said.

"Which nurse?" I queried.

"Hmm. I don't remember," she answered.

Given those sorts of incidents, I started to wonder if perhaps I had an angel posing as a nurse looking out for me. I'm not asserting that was the case, but even the possibility became a comfort to me. And regardless of the physical presence of angels, the most important thing is the realization that God is omnipresent — He's always there, and he cares for us!

Shortly after I was released from hospital, I was able to once again attend a church service, where Dr. Henry Schorr addressed the topic of healing and the role of prayer. He said: "The question is not CAN God heal, but DOES God heal?...If we ask for nothing, we'll get exactly what we asked for." That seems very valid — and an affirmation that it's okay (more than okay!) to ask God for help with our troubles.

Just look at Luke 11:13 for more proof of that. *"Which of you fathers, if your son asks for a fish will give him a snake instead? Or if he asks for an egg, will you give him a scorpion? If you then, though you are evil, know how to give good gifts to your children, how much more will your Father in heaven give the Holy Spirit to those who ask him!"*

Prayer must be a crucial part of the healing process — both prayer by the one who's suffering, and prayer by others.

As Dr. Schorr pointed out in his message that day: "Faith is about giving ourselves over to God's care and knowing He will do what's best."

Even though we may suffer from chronic pain or illness, we can still find peace and meaning in our lives. I particularly like a quote I heard recently, attributed to Mother Teresa:

"Joy is not the absence of pain, but the presence of God."

And for Christians, a big part of our hope comes down to eternal life, without the imperfections of this world, including sickness. As Joni Eareckson writes: "*The Bible indicates that our bodies are temporal. Therefore, my paralysis was temporal. When my focus shifted to this eternal perspective, all my concerns about being in a wheelchair became trivial.*"[13]

Chapter Ten

"Trust in the Lord and do good; dwell in the land and enjoy safe pasture. Delight yourself in the Lord and he will give you the desires of your heart."

Psalm 37:3-4

LIVING WITH CHRONIC ILLNESS

It was a huge triumph to be let out of the hospital — to return to my family and home. And yet, in many ways the battle was just beginning. I had physiotherapy sessions at the hospital twice a week, plus an unbelievable amount of doctors' appointments, whether that was my family doctor, my rheumatologist, my nephrologist, my neurologist, my physiatrist or my eye specialist. Moreover, I was also determined to do a limited amount of journalistic and editing work — my employers had kindly been "holding" my contracts for me when I was in the hospital. I really saw getting back to work — even if it was in a moderate way — as a step back towards my normal life, as well as an intellectual challenge for me.

It's really important to experience mental stimuli other than illness-related matters. When all one really has to think about is aches and pains, and the uncertain future, those thoughts will only grow, and each pain will become that much more obvious.

I tried my best to balance out my "recuperation" period with reading, working, some creative writing, visits from friends and quality time with my family.

Initially, all that was very difficult however, as I was still very weak and rather physically challenged. For instance, while I could manage the stairs in our house (slowly and painfully), there were certain deep or soft chairs I had to avoid, lest I be trapped in them and need someone to pull me off!

The cold and ice of our Canadian winters also meant it was a bit hard for me to get out walking, but along with Adam's nanny (who pushed my little son in his stroller), we were able to gradually increase the distance and speed of our walks. And I signed up for some fitness classes with stretching emphasis, initially taking the city's special "handi-bus" provided to help out physically challenged individuals.

In many ways, I felt like my health efforts — between medical and exercise regimes — was at least a part-time job. And that can be disheartening, especially when one really wants to get back to "normal" life.

As I started to get out again and move among healthy people, I felt more and more that my disease wasn't obvious to others. And while no one confronted me directly, I often thought they wondered why or at least noticed that I'd take the elevator rather than a flight of stairs, or sometimes park in "disabled" parking, even though there was no obvious injury to see on me.

In "*Sick and Tired of Feeling Sick and Tired*," by Paul J. Donoghue and Mary E. Siegel, they write about the challenges of what they call an "invisible" illness. That is, people on the street can't recognize the presence of illness at a glance, and even family and friends may be insensitive to one's fatigue or pain, as there's really nothing to see.

In contrast, most people are more than willing to help out someone who is obviously disabled — whether they are in a wheelchair, or walk with a cane, for instance. However, when someone appears to be "able-bodied," they might not have the same patience — to hold open a door, or to wait for a slow walker, for example.

Donoghue and Siegel write: *"Symptoms common to invisible illnesses are chronic fatigue, chronic pain, memory loss, transient vision disturbances, muscle weakness, bladder urgency, peculiar physical sensations (numbness, 'pins and needles,' hot flashes), skin irritation, intestinal distress and cognitive difficulty. These symptoms do no show up in such a way that makes it obvious to an observer that a person is suffering. Unlike a wound that bleeds or requires stitches, a mending limb that is encased in a cast, or malfunctioning legs that necessitate use of a wheelchair, the symptoms of invisible illnesses have no external evidence of suffering that elicit compassion. Instead the patient often endures suspicion and withdrawal from others. And so, in addition to disturbing, even agonizing and disabling symptoms, the patient of invisible illness suffers, often deeply, from the negative reactions of others. Such reactions frequently lead the patient to confusion, loneliness, self-pity and self-doubt."*[14]

When I was first diagnosed with Lupus, friends and family were enormously sympathetic, sending flowers, offering help, and expressing a willingness to listen. However, over time, I started to feel that the novelty wore off for others, and they viewed my illness and sufferings as merely a matter of fact: "Well, Grace has Lupus, and so she's going to have health problems." I'm not saying the people around me didn't continue to be compassionate — they did; but the outpouring of sympathy and compassion that accompanied my initial diagnosis waned over time.

In the hospital, I remember a nurse taking my temperature, and noting I had a fever, at 38 degrees Celsius. "Well, I guess that's normal for you," she said, after consulting my chart. I silently took exception to that. Yes, perhaps I often ran fevers, but it wasn't "normal" for me, and my suffering wasn't any less real, despite the fact that I've had more fevers than the average person!

I think it may be somewhat easier for others to "accept" a friend's illness than it is for the sick person themselves to do so. And regardless of whether or not a sickness may be habitual, or chronic, others must remember the suffering is still a reality, regardless.

Looking back at the early months after my mid-January release from hospital, I realize that I was still very weak. However, as I continued to regain strength, my optimism rebounded. I was working very hard at my exercises, and I was going to come back to health!

In April, my doctors readjusted some of my medications, hoping to give me a further boost. It may have been a mistake, because my improvements seemed to taper off. I broke out in a skin rash that itched and flaked and made me feel generally unattractive and miserable, as I left clouds of skin behind as I moved or sat on furniture.

My eyelids swelled.

When the rash hit my legs, my ankles and feet swelled up and I couldn't fit in my shoes. The skin on the bottom of my feet cracked and bled and it hurt to walk on them.

While a "rash" seems like a fairly harmless phenomenon, compared to some of the other things that had gone on with me, it too proved to be quite dehabilitating.

In July, it appeared I was doing quite well overall, except for the rash. But by August, blood levels showed my muscle inflammation was once again increasing. I felt okay, and hoped it was just a small fluctuation. But within a couple of weeks, I had my doubts, as I started to weaken. I noticed it was increasingly difficult to get up the stairs. Once again, I needed help to get into Doug's truck. And soon, I found I didn't have the strength to cross my legs without lifting them with my hands.

I realized again that despite my best efforts at exercise and optimism; I was not in control. Within a few days, the disease could flare up and take away my strength, and even my whole way of life.

Sure enough, the next blood tests showed my muscle inflammation had skyrocketed, and to make matters worse, my anaemia was getting severe, robbing me of whatever little energy I may have had.

The elders of my church prayed with me, and several assured me I was regularly in their prayers. How supportive it is to know that others are with me in my journey!

One specialist talked about more chemo — something I deeply feared, both because chemotherapy is very hard on one's body (increasing the risk of certain cancers, for instance) and also because my shorn hair was just starting to thicken up!

It was a frightening time, not merely because I was weaker. Rather, the symptoms — the specific pains and weaknesses — evoked clear memories of how I felt before I "crashed," almost a year ago. That was a huge fear — to return to that helpless state.

All my exercise and efforts seemed virtually meaningless as my strength disappeared. But as hard as the physical setback was, the emotional hit was even more severe. Would I just watch my strength entirely disappear? Would I be back in a wheelchair?

My world quickly shrunk again, as I spent most of my days resting, with almost no energy to do anything. And yet, one day as I lay on my bed, I strongly felt an assurance that this time this wasn't going to be a total crash, an all-out collapse.

Rather, this setback would be brought under control. I'm not saying God told me this audibly, but in a quiet moment, I did feel the assurance and peace that this would turn around.

Another specialist sent me as an outpatient to the hospital for three days in a row to get an intravenous blood product called gamma gobulin (IV-IG). I was surprised to see numerous other people with various muscle problems getting the same treatment — many of them receive it on a monthly basis.

The night after my first day of treatment, I found that I could, with effort, cross my legs again, without using my hands. It seemed like a good sign.

Over the next weeks and months my strength continued to improve. Many days I no longer ran fevers. I felt relatively strong, and able to cope with most of the demands of my life, from working, to caring for Adam.

Then, I became increasingly aware that my vision in my right eye seemed to show blurry spots. I went off to eye specialists who attributed it to Lupus, and increased my steroids. Then, the opinion was reversed — I was told it was a retinal infection called toxoplasmosis — probably activated not only by a wacky immune system, but by the volumes of immune suppression drugs I'm ingesting.

The blurring in my right eye got so bad that, with that eye alone, I could no longer read or even watch TV. There's a heavy blurred spot directly in my line of vision. Fortunately, I do have two eyes — something I sincerely thank God for — so I'm still able to function, and accomplish the things I need to do in life.

Looking through the blurred spot is very similar to trying to see through really dirty glasses or a bad smear on a contact lens. My specialist tells me that I shouldn't expect to see much improvement in my damaged eye. However, he says the overall viewing experience should eventually be less jarring, as my brain will adapt to minimize the blur — or something along those lines.

He tells me we'll have to closely monitor what's going on with that eye. When I expressed concern for my other eye, he told me it would be "very rare" for it to also be affected, although not impossible.

The attack on my sight was very frightening, because sight is just so crucial. And for me, as a writer, adequate sight is integral to my work, income, and sense of purpose.

While many terrible things have happened to me, in some ways, this eye problem is the worst, because everything else, so far, I've been able to at least partially recover from. Unless there's divine intervention — and I do believe that's more than possible — I can expect to have serious permanent eye damage.

WHO AM I NOW?

Throughout life, I've got a lot of sense of fulfillment from my activities and accomplishments — from getting articles published to playing piano in church bands. And certainly, the physical act of caring for my son has been tremendously rewarding.

However, this illness has, at least at times, robbed me of the ability to participate in these roles. If I can't even lift my son, what kind of mother can I be? If I don't have the strength to commit to a volunteer role, what kind of contribution can I make? If I don't have the health or the sight to write, where does my sense of self-worth come from?

Chronic illness can force us to re-evaluate our sense of self-worth, until we come to understand that our value as an individual is separate from our abilities. Likewise, our value to God has nothing to do with our physical abilities, and everything to do with the state of our souls.

Lorna Casselman's *reflections*:

"I want to commend my daughter for her fight to live and return to not only life but also a quality of life.

It is the nature of this disease to be overtly present from time to time.

I know that Grace will meet those challenges as they come. God will give her the strength to endure. We are also looking to the Lord for a huge miracle of physical health in her life."

"God is our refuge and strength, an ever present help in trouble. Therefore we will not fear..."

Psalm 46:1-2

AND NOW...

I hold my son's hand as he stomps on the snow. He is thrilled to be outside.

Every little dance and shriek proclaims his joy — at being alive, at the wonder of the world around him.

I don't jump and squeal; I just smile at Adam and walk beside him. And yet, I too am so joyful and thankful to be able to move about, to be able to experience special time with friends and family, and to enjoy the wonder of God's creation.

As I write this, I realize all too clearly that I can't foretell the future.

I am doing quite well right now. I feel quite physically strong. My flexibility is fairly good, and I only rarely feel fevered or sick.

But looking ahead, I don't know what sort of health situation I might encounter.

Will it always be a matter of fighting one problem after another? Will I essentially be able to live a relatively normal life? Will I return to a wheelchair and a physically helpless state?

The fact is, I don't know.

I can only put my trust in God for my future, and make the most of the strength, health and opportunities that are given to me each day.

A MIRACLE IN PROGRESS

On my first visit home to my family in Montreal in almost a year, I was disconcerted when a woman at my parents' church walked up to me and said, "You're a miracle, you know."

I muttered something polite, but couldn't help thinking I didn't feel much like a miracle. That morning, I ached in every joint and muscle and shivered with fever.

And yet, regardless of my health situation, now or in the future, I am indeed a miracle — a testament to God's grace and mercy.

I don't know how healthy I'll be tomorrow or next week, or next month.

But today I feel quite strong and well, and am so thankful for that.

Moreover, I'll make an effort to go out and accomplish meaningful tasks, and spend quality time with people close to me. It doesn't help me at all to worry about the future, and there's a surprising freedom to living in the "now" — making the most of my current strength and opportunities, rather than obsessing over what may or may not happen in the future.

All I can do is accept the unalterable, and wonderful, truth — it's in God's hands.

"Praise be to the God and Father of our Lord Jesus Christ, the Father of compassion and the God of all comfort, who comforts us in all out troubles, so that we can comfort those in any trouble with the comfort we ourselves have received from God."

2 Corinthians 1:3-4

APPENDIX

A LAYPERSON'S GUIDE TO LUPUS

So what is Lupus anyhow? It seems to be one of those diseases that many people have heard of (although not everyone!), but most people don't really know what it is. (And some even need to be assured it's not contagious!)

The lack of knowledge about Lupus isn't really surprising, as it's a very strange disease.

Basically, it's an autoimmune disease where a person's immune system attacks other parts of the body. That could be anything from a rash on the skin, to muscle or joint problems, to serious damage to kidneys, the heart or the brain.

Probably the biggest symptom, shared by most Lupus sufferers, is fatigue. A person with Lupus will need to adopt a lifestyle that allows for periods of rest.

When it comes to a diagnosis of Lupus, for many people this apparently can take years, as they present their doctors with a variety of odd symptoms that could be caused by a whole range of other conditions. So it's easy for doctors to misdiagnose a patient if Lupus is involved.

In *Lupus: The Disease with 1000 Faces*, Dr. Jean-Luc Senécal lists eleven criteria that can be used in diagnosing Lupus. If a patient meets at least four of them, Lupus will be diagnosed. (But still, that's not a very precise means of diagnosis!)

The eleven points, simplified, are:

- A "butterfly" rash on the cheeks and over the bridge of the nose.
- A particular sensitivity to sunlight.
- "Discoid" Lupus — basically a scaly raised rash on the face or the body.
- Ulcers in the mouth or nose.
- Arthritis.
- Inflammation of the lining of the lungs.
- Kidney involvement — swelling in the feet and legs could be an indicator of this.
- Seizures or psychosis.
- Blood disorders, such as anaemia.
- A positive ANA (antinuclear antibodies) blood test. Most Lupus patients have a positive ANA, although not everyone with a positive ANA has Lupus.
- Immunologic disorders, evidenced by blood tests, such as a test for anti-native DNA autobodies.[15]

Another sign of Lupus activity is apparently "low grade" fevers — regular reoccurring fevers that indicate the immune system is busy fighting something in the body. (Unfortunately, with Lupus, that means it may be fighting previously healthy organs!)

People with Lupus are encouraged to stay out of direct sunlight, and to wear a strong sunscreen and a hat when outdoors. While not everyone with Lupus experiences sun sensitivity, apparently there is a connection for many between exposure to the sun and "flares" in the disease.

Researchers have also found links between eating alfalfa sprouts or echinacea and Lupus flares, so they should be avoided by anyone diagnosed with Lupus. While echinacea is purported to boost immune systems, that could be the last thing a Lupus patient needs, as Lupus is basically all about already having an overactive immune system.

Most people diagnosed with Lupus have a normal life expectancy. The exceptions generally have to do with people who experience severe organ involvement. That's due to the effectiveness of the drugs used to treat Lupus. Even 20 years ago, a diagnosis of Lupus meant a seriously reduced life expectancy. However, there can also be complications from the medications, particularly prolonged high dosages of steroids.

Today, there's no cure for Lupus, even though there's considerable research going on in this area. Instead, specialists, including rheumatologists (joints), nephrologists (kidneys), neurologists (brains, nerves and muscles) and dermatologists (skin), treat the symptoms.

Often, that involves prescribing a steroid drug called prednisone. It's inexpensive and can be extremely effective at controlling or eliminating a lot of Lupus symptoms. However, prednisone itself has a lot of possibly unpleasant or dangerous side-effects, including sleeplessness, hair growth, water retention, a swollen face, muscle weakness and even osteoporosis. The higher the dose, and the longer a patient is on the drug, the greater risk of serious complications.

However, some patients can find sufficient relief through the use of aspirin, acetaminophen or other non-steroid anti-inflammatory drugs.

And some specialists also prescribe so-called "anti-malarial" drugs such as Plaquenil, which can increase patients' energy and reduce various Lupus symptoms.[16]

In very serious cases of Lupus, doctors may decide that chemotherapy is necessary, such as the drug Cyclophosphamide. However, it has possibly nasty side-effects, ranging from hair loss to stomach cancer. Moreover, while it's suppressing the immune system to protect the rest of the body; the treatment also makes the patient more susceptible to illnesses, such as colds or flu.[17]

Basically, every drug has potential side effects, and the challenge for the doctors is to find a balance where the benefits of drugs given to a patient outweigh current and possibly future side effects.

Of interest, those with Lupus are supposed to avoid stress, as that too can bring on flares. Of course avoiding stress is difficult to do! Still, a healthy lifestyle with good eating habits, plenty of rest and moderate exercise are considered particularly beneficial for people with Lupus.

BIBLIOGRAPHY

Arthur, Kay, "*Lord, Give Me A Heart For You,*" Waterbrook Press, Colorado Springs, 2001.

Donoghue, Paul J. and Mary E. Siegel, "*Sick and Tired of Feeling Sick and Tired,*" W.W. Norton & Company Inc., New York, 1992.

Eareckson, Joni and Joe Musser, "*Joni,*" G.K. Hall, Boston, 1976.

Fox, Michael J. "*Lucky Man,*" Random House Inc., New York, 2002.

Horowitz, Mark and Marietta Abrams Brill, "*Living with Lupus: A comprehensive guide to understanding and controlling lupus while getting on with your life,*" Plume, New York, 1994.

Jevne, Ronna Fay and Alexander Levitan. "*No Time for Nonsense: Self-Help for the Seriously Ill,*" LuraMedia, San Diego, 1989.

Kubler-Ross, Elizabeth, "*On Death and Dying,*" First Collier Books Trade Edition, New York, 1993.

Lahita, Robert G. and Robert H. Philips, "*Lupus: Everything You Need to Know,*" Avery Publishing Group, Garden City Park, NY, 1998.

Noble Topf, Linda, "*You Are Not Your Illness,*" Fireside, New York, 1995.

Permut, Joanna Baumer, "*Embracing the Wolf*," Cherokee Pub. Co., Atlanta, Ga., 1989.

Philips, Robert H. "*Coping with Lupus*," Penguin Putman Inc., New York, 2001.

Senécal, Jean-Luc, "*Lupus: The Disease with 1000 Faces*," Lupus Canada, 1998.

Smith, Ed. "*From the Ashes of My Dreams*," Flanker Press Ltd., St. John's, Nfld., 2002.

Wallace, Daniel, "*The Lupus Book: A Guide for Patients and their Families*," Oxford University Press, London, 2000.

END NOTES

[1] Ed Smith. "*From the Ashes of My Dreams.*" Flanker Press Ltd. St. John's, Nfld. 2002. Page 104.

[2] Casselman, Grace. "*A Hole in the Hedge.*" Napoleon Publishing, Toronto, 2003.

[3] "*A Hole in the Hedge,*" by Grace Casselman, is a young adult novel publised May 2003 by Napoleon Publishing.

[4] StatsCan's population census says Canada's 2001 population is 31.4 million. A Lupus Canada study says Lupus affects more that 50,000 Canadians.

[5] Elizabeth Kubler-Ross. "*On Death and Dying.*" First Collier Books Trade Edition. New York. 1993. Page 8.

[6] Horowitz, Mark and Marietta Abrams Brill. "*Living with Lupus: A Comprehensive Guide to Understanding and Controlling Lupus while getting on with your Life.*" Plume, New York, 1994. Page 9.

[7] Foreword by Bernie S. Siegel. Linda Noble Topf. "*You Are Not Your Illness.*" Fireside, New York, 1995. Page 12.

[8] Linda Noble Topf. "*You Are Not Your Illness.*" Fireside, New York, 1995. Page 43.

[9]Michael J. Fox. "*Lucky Man.*" Random House Inc. New York, 2002. Page 8.

[10] Kay Arthur. *"Lord, Give Me A Heart For You."* Waterbrook Press. Colorado Springs, 2001. Page 28.

[11] Paul J. Donoghue and Mary E. Siegel. "*Sick and Tired of Feeling Sick and Tired.*" W.W. Norton & Company Inc., New York, 1992. Page 208.

[12] Joni Eareckson and Joe Musser. *"Joni."* G.K. Hall. Boston. 1976. Preface.

[13] Joni Eareckson and Joe Musser. *"Joni."* G.K. Hall. Boston. 1976. Page 201.

[14] Paul J. Donoghue and Mary E. Siegel. "*Sick and Tired of Feeling Sick and Tired.*" W.W. Norton & Company Inc., New York, 1992. Page 4.

[15] Senécal, Jean-Luc. *"Lupus: The Disease with 1000 Faces."* Lupus Canada, 1998. Page 12-13.

[16] Wallace, Daniel J. *"The Lupus Book: A Guide for Patients and their Families."* Oxford University Press. 2000. Page 208.

[17] *"The Lupus Book,"* Page 219.

About the Author

Grace Casselman lives in Calgary, Alberta, along with her husband Douglas and son Adam. She works as a professional freelance journalist covering technology and business issues and also writes novels for young adults — her first novel is: "*A Hole in the Hedge*." Her Web site is at *www.casselman.net* and she welcomes e-mail at *grace@casselman.net.*

Printed in the United Kingdom
by Lightning Source UK Ltd.
108243UKS00001B/33

9 781592 866939